The Butterfly Children

D1461903

**This book is to be returned on or before
the last date stamped below.**

18-10-4

To all the children and young people who have shared their difficulties and pain with us, and who have taught us so much, and to all our colleagues in the multidisciplinary team without whom this work could not be done.

For Churchill Livingstone:

Editorial Director, Health Sciences: Mary Law
Project Manager: Valerie Burgess/Ewan Halley
Project Development Editor: Valerie Dearing
Design: Judith Wright
Illustrator: Tim Smith
Indexer: Tarrant Ranger Indexing
Sales Promotions Manager: Hilary Brown

The Butterfly Children
An Account of Non-directive Play Therapy

Carole Kaplan MB ChB FRCPsych

Senior Lecturer, Department of Child Health, University of Newcastle upon Tyne
Consultant in Child and Adolescent Psychiatry, City Health NHS Trust,
Newcastle upon Tyne, UK

Rick Telford DipCOT DipDTh

Head Occupational Therapist and Senior Lecturer in Occupational Therapy,
City Health NHS Trust, Newcastle upon Tyne, and the University of Northumbria,
Coach Lane Site, Newcastle upon Tyne, UK

Foreword by
Lily I. H. Jeffrey FCOT UCCAP

Occupational Manager, West Lothian NHS Trust, Livingston, UK
Formerly Head Occupational Therapist, Nuffield Child Psychiatry Unit and
Honorary Occupational Therapy Tutor, University of Newcastle upon Tyne, UK

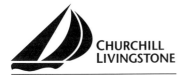

CHURCHILL
LIVINGSTONE

EDINBURGH LONDON NEW YORK PHILADELPHIA SYDNEY AND TORONTO 1998

CHURCHILL LIVINGSTONE
An imprint of Harcourt Brace and Company Limited

© Harcourt Brace and Company Limited 1998

First published 1998

ISBN 0443 054681

British Library Cataloguing in Publication Data
A catalogue record for this book is available from the British Library.

Library of Congress Cataloging in Publication Data
A catalogue record for this book is available from the Library of Congress.

Medical knowledge is constantly changing. As new information becomes available, changes in treatment, procedures, equipment and the use of drugs become necessary. The editors/authors/contributors and the publishers have, as far as it is possible, taken care to ensure that the information given in this text is accurate and up to date. However, readers are strongly advised to confirm that the information, especially with regard to drug usage, complies with the latest legislation and standards of practice.

The
publisher's
policy is to use
**paper manufactured
from sustainable forests**

Printed in China

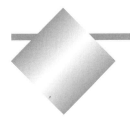

Contents

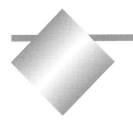

Foreword

Newcastle upon Tyne has a proud history of health services for children. Over the past 50 years, in social paediatrics and in child and adolescent mental health, eminent research has enabled services for children to be planned, organized and developed on evidence-based practice. Underpinning this academic excellence are clinicians dedicated to delivering high-quality services to alleviate childrens' illness, trauma, disability and distress.

In 1967, the Nuffield Child Psychiatry Unit (now the Fleming Nuffield Unit), with facilities for in-patients, replaced the Tiverlands Day Unit. Professor Issy Kolvin, in cooperation with his consultant colleagues, worked tirelessly to create a child mental health resource which was based on a true multidisciplinary environment. In the Unit, all disciplines, including occupational therapy, were encouraged to develop creative new approaches to help disturbed children and establish postgraduate education and training. This book is one of the fruits of that creativity.

Non-directive play therapy, the model of therapy chosen to help the child described in this book, was devised by Virginia Axline half a century ago (Axline 1989). Axline's eight basic principles of therapy seem simplistic in comparison with the sophisticated approaches to therapy today, yet they are essential elements for creating a sound therapeutic space for any patient. Within this secure, supportive, therapeutic environment emotional health can develop. However, the authors of this book indicate that it is in the context of the psychodynamic therapeutic relationship forged between child and therapist that the therapy occurs. They outline a variety of development models and psychodynamic theory to illustrate how intrapsychic change takes place.

Books such as this one and *Dibs: In Search of Self* (Axline 1971) make it seem almost as if the development of that therapeutic relationship and subsequent therapy can be achieved with ease. These books are written by experienced therapists with therapeutic knowledge and skills, who know the importance of creating a therapeutic space for the disturbed child. Therapists engaged in this type of work will readily acknowledge the difficulties of 'holding' the child's emotional pain, anger, frustrations and fears. This book clearly illustrates the importance of support for the therapist by providing regular clinical supervision. Supervisors must themselves be skilled in this type of work. Hawkins and Shohet (1989) have described good supervision in terms of the 'therapeutic triad', i.e. the supervisor supporting and 'holding' the feelings of therapist and child to allow therapy to progress.

This book outlines the essential factors for good multidisciplinary teamwork in the therapeutic milieu of the in-day-patient unit, where the child's named nurse and teacher are key figures. Role clarification is essential so that all team members can contribute their own unique skills to the child's overall treatment. The book illustrates the resources needed to treat children with these types of difficulties and the time needed for effective change to take place.

The Butterfly Children is a valuable addition to child mental health litera-ture. In this decade, society has become acutely aware of the plight of abused children, whether the abuse is emotional, physical or sexual. This book presents a practical approach to play therapy for such children, interspersed with relevant theory.

Who should read this book? First, therapists of all disciplines who use the play medium as a form of therapy. It is important that child psychia-trists, paediatricians and general practitioners are aware of how such interventions can help emotionally disturbed children. Teachers, social workers and those involved in the legal process will find the book invaluable as it clearly illustrates how these traumatized children view their confusing world. Last, and certainly not least, clinical directors and managers who are responsible for resources, to enable them to see that cost-effective intervention at an early stage in a child's life can alleviate distress which if untreated would result in greater costs to society in adolescence and adulthood.

The most important people to benefit from this book will be the disturbed children who require this type of intervention. This type of work is not available for all who need it. To the therapists and their students who provide this type of treatment, the book will be an inspiration to continue their needful work. There can be no greater reward for therapists than to see the personality of their own 'Amber' or 'Dibs' emerge as they make that therapeutic journey from chrysalis to butterfly.

Lily I. H. Jeffrey

REFERENCES

Axline V M 1971 Dibs: in search of self. Penguin Books Ltd, Harmondsworth
Axline V M 1989 Play therapy. Churchill Livingstone, Edinburgh
Hawkins P, Shohet R 1989 Supervision in the helping professions. Open
    University Press, Buckingham

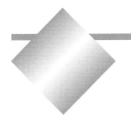

Preface

We have worked together with many children and families referred to our department, and some of the most troubling and difficult problems we have dealt with have concerned children who have been abused. Helping such children is hard and often painful work which can stretch personal and professional resources to the utmost. It can also be very rewarding work and have surprisingly encouraging outcomes. There is little to compare with the joy of seeing a damaged and deeply distressed child emerging from a time of darkness and chaos as an individual willing to tackle whatever the future holds with resourcefulness. One of our patients compared herself to a butterfly emerging from a chrysalis and this book is named *The Butterfly Children* as a tribute to her and other children like her.

The book is based on a case history of one child, Amber. 'Amber' is, in fact, a composite of many children we have known and worked with, all with their own particular strengths. We hope this account demonstrates the optimism and resilience children can show in the face of such traumatic experiences, as well as the periods of hope and despair which professionals must deal with when trying to help them. This case history is used both to demonstrate the techniques and tensions of working together as professionals and to demonstrate the effectiveness of this form of non-directive play therapy.

The idea for this book arose a long time ago and the writing of it has occurred in several countries. We would like to thank our families for their support and encouragement throughout this time, especially Peter, James, Sarah and Lynn. We would also like to remenber those members of our families who, sadly, did not live to see the finished book.

Newcastle 1998

Carole Kaplan
Rick Telford

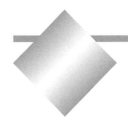

The structure of the book

The account in this book follows a chronological sequence, from the initial referral and assessment, through the discussions and interactions with other agencies, to the therapy, which is described in detail and ends with Amber's last visit to the unit at Christmas time.

A chapter on the issues relating to the legal context of this work has been included (Ch. 6). The Children Act 1989, for England and Wales, is the context in which we work, but the bulk of the chapter deals with general principles of assessment and court work, providing a more wide-ranging applicability for the professional. Chapter 10 covers the case review at the end of Amber's therapy sessions.

Each chapter has been written with the clinical and therapeutic descriptions first, followed by an account of the discussions between the occupational therapist and child psychiatrist which highlight the theoretical frameworks and seek explanations for Amber's behaviour and emotional responses. These discussions cover different psychodynamic and developmental theories, and focus on the various forms of intervention that can be tried.

General information has been separated from Amber's case study and boxed so that readers can read the case study uninterrupted by teaching points, if they so wish.

Note
As the therapist in this case study is male, all references to the therapist are 'he', and, as Amber is a girl, all references to the child are 'she'.

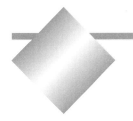

Glossary

Neutral: play used to build a therapeutic relationship.

Regressive: the child uses play at a level below that expected for her chronological age and intellectual endowment because it satisfies an emotional need.

Aggressive: activity used to express aggression.

Projective: play used by the child to communicate feelings, fears and fantasies.

Fantasy: representational play using themes which imitate adult activities.

Social: cooperative play between children.

Constructive: purposeful use of play materials or toys.

Creative: a child's unique influence on play materials.

Directed play: structured use of the play situation by the therapist.

1

Meeting the family

Referrals

The child psychiatry and psychology department receives referrals from general practitioners, social services departments, schools and education services, hospital and community-based paediatricians, and other psychiatrists and psychologists. Referrals are also accepted from the legal services for the purpose of providing expert opinions for the courts. Many regional centres have in-patient and/or day-patient units as well as active out-patient clinics within the hospital and in the community. Children and families are seen if they are referred because of concerns about a wide range of emotional and behavioural problems, some of which will be diagnosed as formal psychiatric disorders. A large number of therapeutic interventions, including individual therapy, family therapy, group therapy, behaviour and drug therapy, are available in a combination of settings after assessment.

THE INITIAL REFERRAL

On a busy day in September, the child psychiatrist received a letter from the local social services department which asked if she would see 7-year-old Amber and her family. The letter stated that the social worker was worried about Amber because she had arrived at school with a big bruise on her temple. This had been found at a time when the teachers had been concerned about Amber's inappropriately intrusive behaviour towards other children over a number of months. When the teacher had asked Amber's mother about the bruise she had said that Amber had fallen and banged her head on a table and had become very withdrawn. Later that day, Amber had been found masturbating in the toilets in full view of other children.

There had been concern about Amber for some time, because she was pale and small for her age, and often had bumps and bruises for which she and her mother gave a variety of explanations. The social worker was also concerned about Amber's brother and sister, who were also both small for their age. Jenny, who was 3 years old, was seldom heard to speak and Craig, aged 5 years, was said to be difficult to manage at school and had been described as 'hyperactive.' The school staff were concerned that Amber did not seem to make friends easily and was 'mostly on the edges of the other children's groups.' Her work was very poor, she lacked concentration, and was either hostile or unresponsive to the teachers.

The social worker explained that many attempts had been made to talk to the children's mother, Katherine. However, this had proved to be difficult as she was often not in at agreed appointment times, or refused to discuss any concerns about her children on the basis that they were her responsibility and no one had any business to interfere in how she cared for them. In the social worker's view, the family seemed isolated in the community.

A report from a consultant paediatrician was also enclosed. It described a thin, quiet child, short and light for her age, with five bruises of different ages on her arms, legs and forehead. Amber had said that her 'tuppence was sore' and examination of her genitalia had shown signs suggestive of penetrative sexual abuse. When told of the paediatrician's findings Amber's mother had said Amber often 'played with herself' or rubbed her genital area against objects, such as the arm of a chair or part of her bicycle. She added that Amber could not have been sexually abused as she always looked after the children herself, or else a good friend, whom she had known for years, babysat on the rare occasions when she went out.

As a result of the findings, and in the light of the longstanding concern about the family, the three children had been taken into care by the social services department and an interim care order had been granted by the court. In addition, Amber had been interviewed by the police on video, with the support of a social worker, in order to try to gain further information about the alleged child abuse. Amber had said that someone had shouted at her and hit her and added that Alan (Katherine's partner) had 'hurt my tuppence.' After this disclosure she had curled up and refused to talk or play any further.

In many situations where child abuse is suspected the evidence may not be very substantial. In this case, there was concern about physical growth and development, progress at school, peer relationships, and behaviour. There was a 'disclosure' or allegation by the child, and the only 'evidence' was the discovery, on physical examination, of bruises and signs suggestive of penetrative sexual abuse. In many similar situations, the physical evidence may be even more equivocal and there may be no allegation at all. It can be very difficult in these circumstances to know whether abuse has taken place or not and it is essential for professionals to keep an open mind, while taking the child's statement seriously. For a prosecution to be considered a suspect is needed and, often, while it is agreed that abuse has occurred, the perpetrator is unknown.

The objectives of the assessment

The assessment is usually completed by a psychiatrist or psychologist, working alone or with other members of the multidisciplinary team. The process generally includes interviews with the child, her parents and siblings, and other significant individuals, such as grandparents and foster parents. The objectives of assessment are threefold:

1. To assess the child's level of functioning in terms of emotional, social and cognitive abilities, as well as her mental state and areas of vulnerability and resilience.

2. To assess suitability for therapeutic intervention and to determine the kind of therapy that would be most appropriate.

3. To prepare a report for the referring agent , which may be the court, which deals with a wide range of issues including the needs of the child, any issues of past or potential harm to the child, and also advice as to the possible consequences of a variety of options for future care of the child.

These objectives are more likely to be achieved if the following points are taken into account:

1. Sufficient factual information must be gathered to allow an objective view to be formed of developmental, temperamental and family factors, as well as any life experiences that the child has had.

2. A brief assessment of the child's ability to relate to the interviewer, her use of language, play and drawing skills, and an understanding of her recent experiences, is helpful. A calm, non-judgmental approach, in a setting where the requirements of the adult are clear to the child, is likely to facilitate this. Clearly, this must be done at a level which is appropriate to the child and where the child's needs and reactions are always put first.

3. It is easier for the child if the clinician gives some explanation of what is going to happen, for example, that there will be talking and playing, but no physical examinations or use of needles as these are often associated with hospitals.

4. It is helpful if the clinician tells the child that she knows a little about her, such as where she lives, where she goes to school and any recent major changes in her life, such as moving home.

5. It is very important for the child to have a good experience on her first visit to the department. The knowledge that she is important enough to be listened to carefully, that an adult has devoted time and energy to her alone and is concerned about her needs and wishes, gives a positive message to the child that she is valued. This helps her to feel less apprehensive about returning to the department. A positive perception provides a good foundation on which to build future professional relationships.

AMBER'S ASSESSMENT

Following the referral, an appointment was made for Amber, Jenny and Craig to be seen, together with their foster parents, by the child psychiatrist. The child psychiatrist also arranged to see the children's mother later on the same day.

The foster mother and social worker arrived early with the children (the foster father was unable to attend) and met the out-patient nurse, who offered them a drink while they waited. Craig accepted this and played on the rocking-horse and with the other toys with some enthusiasm. Jenny sat on her foster mother's knee and watched the others. Amber sat alone, bolt upright on a chair, watching her siblings constantly. She made little response to approaches by the nurse and seemed to withdraw even further when Craig approached her to ask her to play with him.

MEETING THE SOCIAL WORKER

The social worker told the child psychiatrist that her department had been concerned about all three of the children since the concerns of the school were made known to them about 2 years previously. She said that she and her colleagues had repeatedly tried to talk to Katherine, the children's mother, about their concerns but she had always been dismissive of them and had always had a plausible explanation for any specific matters, such as marginal weight gain by Jenny or Amber's wetting herself at school and at home. Katherine often said that the children had been ill and when this was checked with the general practitioner or school nurse they had notes stating that the children had had minor illnesses. Until the most recent events, the social services department had not been concerned enough to intervene more actively. The social worker said that she was most concerned about Amber, who was clearly a rather difficult and unusual child, apparently with a limited capacity for understanding quite ordinary questions or situations. It was felt that Amber must be a challenging child to care for as she was so unresponsive and of limited intellectual ability.

Meeting the foster mother

The foster mother, Margaret, said that the children had been brought to her with their belongings in large plastic bags. Each of them had brought a soft toy, apart from Amber who had come empty-handed. Amber had asked where she was to sleep and where her brother and sister were to sleep, and then had obeyed most instructions, such as 'It is time to wash your hands for dinner', in silence. Craig had engaged immediately in play with toys available in the house, and Jenny had attached herself to the foster mother, and refused to leave her side. Over the 6 weeks that the children had been in foster care, Craig's behaviour had become less impulsive and overactive, and Jenny had gradually accepted separation from her foster mother for brief periods, but Amber had remained quiet and unusually obedient. She only spoke when spoken to and the only activities she engaged in spontaneously were tidying her own, Jenny and Craig's beds, and brushing Jenny's hair. All three of the children had settled into a daily routine of school, play, bath and bed, and their physical health seemed to have improved. Jenny and Craig ate voraciously but Amber only ate a little of the food given to her and had not gained any weight, unlike Jenny and Craig.

Margaret told the child psychiatrist that the children saw their mother at the local social services office twice a week. Amber suffered nightmares after these visits and Margaret wondered if they made Amber remember 'bad' things that had happened to her as she often cried out in her sleep or, if she woke, seemed terrified. She said that Amber did not speak intelligibly in her sleep and if Margaret went to comfort her, after she had woken from one of these dreams, she only sobbed. Once she had said her mother's name and asked if her mother was safe. There was no other change in Amber's behaviour apart from the nightmares. The visits also affected the other two children. Jenny returned to her silent, clingy behaviour and Craig became destructive and verbally aggressive. However, they returned to a more usual pattern of behaviour and interactions after a few hours. Margaret said that the children had spent a few hours with their maternal grandfather and his second wife when they visited the foster home. The children had been pleased to see their grandparents but very excitable and difficult to settle for several hours after their departure.

Meeting the children

After talking to the social worker and foster mother, the child psychiatrist went with Margaret to meet Amber, Jenny and Craig. They had been spending time in the waiting room with a member of the nursing staff. Jenny ran to her foster mother and hugged her, asking where she had been. The foster mother explained that she had been 'talking to the nice doctor' and that 'now it was the children's turn' to meet her. Craig stopped playing with the Lego and he and Jenny each took one of their foster mother's hands. Amber got up from her chair and silently followed them to the child psychiatrist's office. This was a well-lit room with a sand tray and many toys to play with. Margaret sat in a comfortable armchair and Jenny sat on her knee; Craig played in the sand tray with cars and soldiers; Amber sat on a small child's chair with a tense upright posture.

The child psychiatrist said that she was a doctor who was interested in children, in what kinds of things they do, how they felt and the many different things that happened to children, some good, some bad. She explained that she tried to help children by trying to understand the sort of things they thought about and also the kinds of feelings they may have. The child psychiatrist added that she was different from some of the other doctors they may have met, as she would not listen to their chests or look in their ears but would rather talk and play with them.

All three of the children listened very carefully to what she said, although Craig continued playing in the sand and Jenny hugged a teddy bear and snuggled into her foster mother's arms. Amber watched the child psychiatrist carefully, seldom taking her eyes from her face and focusing mostly on the child psychiatrist's lips as she talked.

The child psychiatrist asked if anyone had any questions or anything they wanted to say. Craig asked if he could play with another toy and was readily given permission to play with some construction bricks. The doctor said that she knew a little about Amber, Craig and Jenny. She knew that they were living with Margaret, their foster mother, at the moment, but that they used to live with their mother and Alan. She added that she knew that they spent time with their mother twice a week and would see her again the next day and that they had also been visited by their grandfather and grandmother. The child psychiatrist said that she knew that when children went to live with new families it could be very different from what they had been used to and she hoped to be able to try to understand what this was like for each of them. To do this she would need to see them again. Craig interrupted at this point and asked if he could come the next day, and was reassured that arrangements would be made for him and Jenny and Amber to come again. The session ended with cheerful farewells from Craig and Jenny, and a solemn 'Goodbye, doctor' from Amber.

Meeting the mother

The purpose of meeting the parents

It is important to meet the parents of children being assessed as firstly they have parental responsibility for the child, even if this may be shared with others, and secondly they can give important information about the child's conception, gestation and birth. The parents can also provide information about their own backgrounds which can have an important effect on how they relate to their own children and how they have provided parental care for the child. The parents can also talk about their relationship with each other and their perception of the relationship between the other parent and the children. Vital information about the child's early life experiences and developmental course can be gathered from the parents as well as concerns about, and perceptions of, the child.

Katherine, the children's mother, was a tall, slender, dark-haired woman in her late twenties. She was fashionably dressed and had a very assertive manner. She said that she was very annoyed that she had been forced to come and that neither she nor her children needed to see a psychiatrist. When asked why she thought the children had been referred by the social worker she said that it was 'all because of a small bruise on Amber's forehead' and because an 'interfering paediatrician' said that Amber had been sexually abused. Katherine stated emphatically that this was not true and anything that may have been seen in Amber's 'privates' were as a result of her rubbing herself. She commented that Amber often rubbed herself on the arm of a chair or part of her bike. Katherine said that she was perfectly capable of looking after her children and that 'people should not be interfering where they are not wanted or needed.'

The child psychiatrist asked Katherine if she had any worries or concerns about either Amber, Jenny or Craig. She said that she had been worried about Amber rubbing at herself but other than that she had no concerns or 'nothing for a child psychiatrist or social worker to be worried about anyway.' When asked to expand on this, Katherine said that Amber and Craig were not doing very well at school and that

Amber's work in particular had deteriorated in the last term. Katherine said that she felt that this was because Amber had difficulty changing schools and also because she had had a lot of chest infections during the autumn. Craig was 'very naughty' at school and the teacher had asked Katherine to come in and talk to her about him next week. She said she was 'sure it was nothing serious.' The child psychiatrist pointed out to Katherine that she knew there had been concerns on the part of the school for some time and she also knew that the paediatrician had found physical evidence suggestive of sexual abuse. Katherine said that it was impossible that Amber had been sexually abused and she was certain that the physical signs were as a result of Amber rubbing at herself and nothing else.

When the interview ended Katherine returned to the waiting room where the children had been sitting and playing with a member of the nursing staff. Craig and Jenny greeted their mother fairly neutrally, whereas Amber ran to her and clung to her, repeatedly asking Katherine if she was all right. With some encouragement and a degree of firmness from their mother, Jenny and Craig stopped playing with the toys and the family left, the children with their foster mother. Katherine left by herself, after giving each child a hug, which Amber initially tried to prolong and then ended by letting go abruptly.

The second meeting with the mother

The purpose of the interviews with the mother

Information about the mother's personal history provides an insight into her own experiences as a child and the kind of parental care that she received. Her ability to form relationships and her perceptions of the role and style of parents can be greatly influenced by her experiences as a child herself, in both a conscious and unconscious way. Information about any physical or psychiatric illnesses or difficulties on the mother's part can indicate additional vulnerabilities the child has to deal with. An account of the mother's adult experiences of employment, relationships and other life events can add significantly to an understanding of her capacity to care for her children and the vicissitudes the children may have had to cope with. Just as important is an understanding of the good experiences of parenting and the positive aspects of relationships between the mother and the children.

On the next occasion that Katherine came to the child psychiatry department she wore a long black skirt and a black blouse, and a lot of jangling silver jewellery and bright make-up. Once again she adopted an assertive manner and repeated that she had only come because 'it would look bad to the court if I didn't.' Once the child psychiatrist had said that she was glad to have the opportunity to talk to her again, she became more cooperative and agreed to give her an account of her personal history, on the basis that if the child psychiatrist knew her better she 'would realise that the accusations were nonsense.' Katherine talked about her 'ordinary happy childhood' while her parents remained together with her and her brother John until she was 8 years old. She said that after that there was a lot of fighting between her parents, ending with her father deserting the family. Katherine recalled school and further training as positive experiences where she succeeded in gaining skills and recognition which she had not been offered at home.

Katherine said that when she finished school she left home for good as a result of the poor relationship she had with her mother's new partner who used to hit her and her brother. She recalled a number of short-lived relationships with men, in which she felt they had used her only for sexual gratification, or to provide them with money or somewhere to live 'but none of them really bothered about me as a person.' She said that she began to drink heavily and started to use amphetamines and barbiturates on a regular basis. She became pregnant with Amber unexpectedly and continued to use these substances throughout this and her other two pregnancies. She was not absolutely certain who the father of each child was but recalled that she 'never told anyone anyway.' Amber was born in hospital by normal vertex delivery, after very little antenatal care, with a birth weight of 6lbs 3 ozs (2.8 kg). Katherine said that the labour was long and difficult and they were worried about Amber's heartbeat being too slow.

After delivery Amber had been kept in the special care baby unit as she was jaundiced and she did not feed well. Katherine said, 'In the end they stuck a tube into her arm and they fed her through it, but it kept coming out and she was a mass of bruises where they kept putting new ones in. Amber cried all the time and hardly slept. They kept wanting me to be with her but I was exhausted. I needed some drugs and I couldn't stand her crying so much.'

Katherine recalled how she had been alone for the delivery and had to care for Amber alone. A similar pattern of conception and abandonment was described for Jenny and Craig, but Katherine emphasised her resilience and ability to cope despite adversity. Katherine said that she had found Amber to be a 'whingy, whiney baby' who had irritated her. She had often left her with various friends who had children of their own and 'were good mothers.' She had continued to use drugs regularly and had worked sporadically to pay for this. She said she had never been incapable of work or caring for her children because of the drugs. Katherine formed a relationship which had lasted for 4 years with Alan, an attractive man with a university degree who used to deal in drugs. She said that 'the police and other dealers were always after him and I was afraid but he said it was OK.' Katherine said that Alan used to sometimes get very angry with Amber but denied he ever hit her. She said their flat was always full of people ('the kids enjoyed this, there were lots of things going on') and added that the group of adults did use drugs together 'for recreational purposes' but the children were asleep when this happened.

Amber had gone to the local nursery and infant school and the teachers had always said she was a solitary, quiet child who behaved oddly sometimes. In class she was 'behind with her work' and there were times when she seemed 'not all there.' Katherine emphasized that she had frequently asked for help with Amber but this had never been provided by the authorities. She said that her father had kept in touch and 'every now and again he sent presents to the kids or took them out for a hamburger.' She added that he always seemed critical of how she cared for the children and 'we used to argue and he came less often.'

The second meeting with Amber

The purpose of the interviews with the child

During the interviews with the child it is important to gain the trust of the child sufficiently to allow her to communicate. The clinician aims to try to get some understanding of the child's developmental level, her language and understanding, and her sense of the world around her. It is very important to proceed at the child's pace and not to drive forward to try to complete set tasks in a short space of time. With some children, it may take a number of interviews before the clinician feels that she has adequate information to comment on any of these aspects of a child's functioning. For a child psychiatrist, a mental state examination will also be done to establish whether the child is suffering from any formal mental illness, but this is done as informally and unintrusively as possible so that it forms a natural part of an interaction with a child.

In addition to establishing some form of assessment, the child must be helped to interact with the clinician in such a way as to facilitate future relationships with therapists and other professionals. Thus the child must be made to feel that she has been listened to carefully, that what she does and says is important, and that she is given adequate time, space and attention to allow her to communicate what she can or needs to tell.

Amber came to see the psychiatrist again on a wet and windy day. She was neatly dressed in a navy skirt and blue jumper, looking oddly old fashioned for her age. The dark rings under her eyes stood out sharply in her pale thin face and her short, thin hair had little life. She accompanied the child psychiatrist to her office without comment and sat on the edge of her chair, with the child psychiatrist sitting a little away from her on a low chair to her side. Once again she fixed her eyes on the child psychiatrist's face as she asked Amber how she had come to the unit and with whom. There was silence as the child psychiatrist waited for her replies but none came. The child psychiatrist talked of the last time they had met and recalled some of the things she had said to Amber. She reminded Amber that she had said that one of the things that they could do together was to play a game, or they could draw.

Without speaking Amber nodded and moved slowly to a table where she selected a floor puzzle of fishes under the sea. The child psychiatrist helped her to put it on the floor and unpack it. Amber then sat in silence, apparently not understanding what the large coloured pieces of card were for. When the child psychiatrist asked her to help turn the jigsaw pieces over so that the coloured sides were uppermost, Amber slowly did this, looking at her for confirmation that she was doing the right thing, only turning over the next piece when she had quietly been given assurance that she was doing well.

Slowly, and almost without talking, the adult and child gradually fitted some of the pieces of the puzzle together. Once some of the fishes became identifiable the child psychiatrist remarked on the bright colours and Amber nodded and said, 'That one is yellow', and completed that part of the jigsaw alone. In a quiet voice she then added, 'It must be nice there', and, after an encouraging, 'Mmmmm', from the child psychiatrist added, 'It's windy here. It was raining when we came from Margaret's house.' The child psychiatrist smiled at her and together they finished the jigsaw.

Amber seemed unable to decide what she wanted to do next so the child psychiatrist asked if she could talk to her a little, to which Amber agreed. She began by checking Amber's age, which school she went to and the name of her teacher. Amber gave this information slowly and seemed uncertain of the name of the school and her teacher. The child psychiatrist remarked that she knew that some people liked school and others didn't and she wondered what Amber thought about school. There was no reply to this and Amber appeared not to understand what had been said, turning toward the doll's house instead.

Amber and the child psychiatrist opened the house together and then the child psychiatrist sat back as Amber took out each of the tiny dolls and examined them carefully. She then looked at the furniture, took a baby's cot and tried to push one of the larger girl dolls into it. When she would not fit, Amber commented that it was too big and rapidly pushed it, and the other dolls and all the furniture, back into the house very roughly and forced the house shut. She then went to sit in a big chair and looked out of the window. The child psychiatrist said that she had been glad to talk to Amber and to look at the dolls and the doll's house with her, and that they would meet again. Amber asked if she could see into the doll's house again before she went and after she had done this, and shown the child psychiatrist that there was a big mess inside, she returned quietly to her foster mother.

Observations on the second meeting

In each succeeding meeting, it is important to acknowledge to the child that the clinician remembers what happened before and also remembers any assurances that were given to the child. The idea that the child communicates through play as well as verbal exchanges is crucial to this form of work. A child able to tell the child psychiatrist of the mess in her home, perhaps reflecting that in her mind, as directly as was done in the session described, is unusual. It is far more common for a child to show tiny things slowly in the gradual process of forming a relationship.

It must be remembered that this section of work is assessment not therapy and so the relationship will necessarily be fairly superficial. However, it is of great importance that a good model of interaction is given to the child to facilitate further therapeutic work.

The third meeting with Amber

On the third meeting, Amber went straight to the sea jigsaw, put it on the floor, sat down next to it and looked at the child psychiatrist, who said, 'I think you want me to do the jigsaw with you?' Amber nodded and said quietly, 'We did it last time', to which the child psychiatrist nodded and said, 'You liked the colours', and helped set out the pieces.

Amber tried to fit some of these together but could not get this right and would not tolerate any help. She leaned back and said, 'No', and curled into a small ball, sucking her finger. The child psychiatrist observed that sometimes it was hard to do things and that could make people sad and angry. There was no response to this and Amber remained curled up.

The child psychiatrist remained sitting on the floor next to Amber, and after a little while Amber turned a little towards her and said, 'I cry sometimes, so does my Mum.' The child psychiatrist said that everyone cried from time to time and that was fine. Amber said that she knew that her brother and sister cried sometimes 'but not like me' and curled up tightly again. The child psychiatrist said that sometimes she must feel very lonely and Amber gave a fleeting nod. After a while Amber stood up and asked to paint. She made a squiggly pattern which she coloured green and brown and said that she would like to give this to her mother because 'she misses me and she likes green.' The child psychiatrist agreed to this and carefully they rolled the picture up and put a rubber band around it. Amber then said, 'Maybe I will see this again when I go home,' and began to suck her thumb and rock gently in her chair. Then suddenly she leapt to her feet, picked up the rolled picture, tore it several times and threw it to the floor. Amber turned in a frightened way toward the child psychiatrist who said calmly, 'You seemed to be angry when you threw the picture onto the floor. That is all right.' Amber hid her face in her hands and her thin body shook as she cried silently. She accepted a tissue from the child psychiatrist whom she allowed to sit near to her and then she suddenly stopped crying. She asked if they could tidy up and together the adult and child picked up the pieces of paper and put them in an envelope, which Amber put in the back of her casenotes.

After sitting quietly for a short time the child psychiatrist said that it was the end of their time together and Amber got up, said, 'See you again,' waited for the reply, 'Yes, you will,' and returned to her foster mother.

The final assessment meeting

It is very important for a child to know what will happen in assessment sessions: where they will be and how long they will last, the kinds of activities that might be done, and how many there will be. It is necessary to help the child to trust the person doing the assessment, but care must be taken that the child is aware that there will be only a few such meetings and what their purpose is. The child must receive the message that all that she conveys is important, that different ways of expressing emotion are acceptable provided that they are reasonably safe, and that there is an unconditional acceptance of the child.

The final meeting with Amber

At the final meeting, the child psychiatrist reminded Amber that they had met three times and that today was the last time they would meet and talk and play in this way. She then went on to say that they had done a number of things together and Amber helped her to list the jigsaws, games and pictures they had used. Amber said, 'Last time you picked up the pieces of paper and I put them away.' The child psychiatrist nodded and showed Amber that the envelope containing the pieces was still there. The child psychiatrist went on to say that there had been a lot of different feelings when they had spent time together, and she thought that at times Amber had felt sad, lonely and also cross. Amber agreed and said, 'But sometimes it was all right,' and added, 'It rained when I first came here.'

The child psychiatrist listened and then said that she knew that there were a lot of difficult things for Amber to think about , and she wondered if it might help to have someone to listen to her and play with her, and to try to help her to understand what was happening so that one day things might feel a little easier for her. Amber thought about this for several minutes then went to the doll's house. She took each doll and all the furniture out before putting them all back very carefully, but she put the beds in the kitchen, the car in the bedroom, and tables and chairs in the garage. She then closed the house firmly and asked, 'Will I come here again?' The child psychiatrist replied that she would come to the same place but would not spend time with her but rather with a colleague. Amber said, 'No, I want to see you,' but when it was explained that this was not possible, as she needed to see someone who could be there every week who was particularly good at helping children, she agreed on condition that she saw the child psychiatrist sometimes, which the child psychiatrist said she could.

2

The team meeting

Team meetings

At a team meeting, the details of a case are described and advice and opinions are sought from all the members of the multidisciplinary group. The team consists of nurses, therapists, social workers, teachers, psychologists and psychiatrists. The philosophy behind a multidisciplinary approach is that bringing together different people, with different training and experience as well as differing viewpoints, aids the understanding of difficult problems. It also helps to plan future management and intervention, if any is required. Usually, the team will have worked together for some time and faced some complex issues together, therefore, the discussions take place in an atmosphere of trust and respect which allows for full, and sometimes conflicting, views to be put forward. The team based in the hospital also works closely with professionals in the community. In Amber's case, this meant working with the social worker based in the community and regular communication, sharing and joint planning with the social worker, if needed, on a daily basis.

At the meeting, the child psychiatrist described the problems with which Amber had been referred, described her home background, and referred to the particular concerns of the social worker (which the social worker later amplified). The child psychiatrist said that her initial formulation was that Amber was a 7-year-old child who presented with behaviour problems consisting of withdrawal, inappropriate sexualized behaviour, nightmares, and soiling and wetting. Physical examination suggested the possibility of physical and sexual abuse and also raised concerns about physical growth and development. Intellectually, Amber had been maintained in mainstream education but her cognitive ability required assessment as she seemed to have difficulty understanding simple instructions and her classwork was below the level expected for her age. Amber had been living with her mother and Alan, her partner for the last 4 years, and her siblings Jenny and Craig. Since the case conference held to consider concerns about child protection, all three children had been in care but with regular contact with their mother. Their legal position was that the social services department had an interim care order for all the children.

The child psychiatrist said that, in her view, Amber was not suffering from a formal psychiatric disorder but that she had difficulties in a range of domains of functioning which were likely to be best explained in terms of reaction to life experiences. The problems Amber was facing included the serious one of abuse, as well as the nature of her relationship with her mother and her siblings. The team needed to try to understand Amber's strengths and vulnerabilities, and work out why she was behaving in such a strange manner at school, with her foster mother, and with her mother. The true level of her ability and resilience needed to be established and a strategy devised to try to help this very needy little girl to see a future for herself.

A lengthy discussion followed as to what factors could have contributed to the way in which Amber was presenting. Such a discussion looks at the effects of both nature (i.e. the child's inherent attributes) and nurture (i.e. the child's environment) on the child. In Amber's case, the prenatal history of deprivation, stress and drug abuse in her mother's life was likely to be a significant factor (Davenport 1989). The development of children exposed to drugs in utero is affected after delivery. Poor nutrition and high levels of stress during pregnancy can also have an adverse effect on development. The team wondered whether Amber's apparent cognitive difficulties could have originated in these antenatal experiences.

Another factor to be considered was the history of a difficult delivery and concern about possible fetal distress. Amber had needed special care on arrival and her period in the special care unit had been difficult both for her and her mother. Katherine had described herself as being exhausted and suffering from an absence of drugs so the early formation of a bond between mother and child was likely to have been troubled.

The fact that Amber had often been left in the care of a large number of different people in her early years, many of whom frequently used drugs, confirmed the view that her early experiences probably included a large amount of uncertainty and anxiety particularly in relation to her attachment to her mother. A child needs to experience constant, reliable parental care from at least one person and this was conspicuously absent in what was known of Amber's early life. Amber's own temperament may have compounded these difficulties. The interactions between children and parents are mediated by the personality or temperament each brings to the relationship. Amber was described as having been a difficult, demanding child who cried frequently and her mother found her difficult to be with. How much of this difficult behaviour was part of Amber's character and how much was due to the questionable care she received was unknown. The interaction of a child with a difficult temperament and a mother who also has difficulties with interpersonal relationships can also be a negative experience for both child and parent caught in this difficult cycle.

The team considered how far the basic needs of a child to be cared for physically, in terms of feeding, cleaning, bathing and being kept warm and safe, were being met. Meeting psychological needs for love and attention, as well as the need to have strong emotions such as rage, despair, hatred and love contained, is also essential. Consistency of care from an identified carer is also needed. The meeting of these needs would have been significantly affected by Katherine's continued heavy use of drugs which at times rendered her incapable of caring for her children properly. From a developmental perspective, this meant that Amber had difficulty establishing a sense of basic trust according to

Erikson's explanation of personality development (Erikson 1965). As a result, she was likely to experience difficulty in forming future relationships if she did not have the opportunity to develop trust. There was evidence that Katherine had difficulty establishing stable relationships and her ability to relate to Amber would have been affected by her own turbulent childhood. She had had many different relationships, some of them characterized by violence, and this unsettled lifestyle would also have added to Amber's insecurity.

The effect of the abuse that Amber had suffered also had to be examined. In her case, it seemed to be physical, sexual and emotional, with her physical and psychological growth affected as well as her behaviour and emotional responsiveness. Amber had shown sexual disinhibition, aggression, and seemed 'switched off' in some areas of functioning in a way that was not consistent or predictable. It was impossible to sort out which experiences may have led to which reactions.

The team identified several areas on which to focus. These were Amber's:

• ability to cope with daily living
• peer and adult relationships
• sense of herself as an individual
• cognitive and educational ability
• relationship with other members of her family.

It was agreed that constitutional, pre-birth and environmental experiences were all likely to have had an impact on Amber. She was seen as a very distressed and traumatized little girl about whom more information was needed in order to produce a more sophisticated formulation to refine the treatment and intervention strategy. The child psychiatrist reminded the team that a formal report for the court would need to be prepared.

The team decided that a period of day-patient attendance, probably extending over several months, was the best way forward. During this time Amber would receive support, education, socialization and care from staff trained and experienced in all aspects of child mental health, at a place with particular experience in helping abused children. The child psychiatrist agreed to seek consent for this from Amber, the social services department and Amber's mother. The next step was to organize a preadmission meeting.

THE PREADMISSION MEETING

The preadmission meeting was held in the unit and was attended by the foster mother and social worker as well as members of the multidisciplinary team who would be working with Amber during her admission. The child psychiatrist outlined Amber's history and gave a description of her impression of Amber and how her difficulties had arisen. The written report sent from the school was discussed. Prior to the meeting Amber had been visited at home by the nurse who would be specially allocated to her and by the class teacher who would work with her in the unit. Following this Amber, her foster mother and the social worker had visited the unit, looked around at the various facilities Amber would be using and met members of staff. Katherine had been invited to all of these events but, although she had telephoned to say she would attend, she had not appeared at any of them. Information from these preadmission visits was shared and discussed and the date and time of admission fixed for the following Monday.

The preadmission meeting

A preadmission meeting is always held before an admission and is part of the planned admission policy. The purpose of the meeting is to ensure that key staff and colleagues from outside the unit have all the relevant information and to ensure that good communication is started, setting the pattern for further close working together. It provides a visible continuity from out-patient to day-patient care, and allows professionals and parents to focus on issues that need to be addressed and to plan an assessment and treatment package to start immediately.

The visits to the home allow the child to meet staff members on her home territory and to begin to form a relationship with people who will be there to greet her and help her to integrate into the unit. Practical issues, such as dietary requirements or preferences, can be discussed, permission obtained to take the child swimming and on other outings if appropriate, and a general description of the unit routine given. Transport, either by the parents or other agency, or by hospital transport in the form of a taxi or minibus, is arranged.

The nurse and teacher who had visited Amber described a child who seemed cut off from ordinary human contact. She was politely present physically and made appropriate responses but emotional reactions were curiously absent and there was no sense of warmth, shyness or curiosity about her impending admission. Amber had complied with all requests but had not seemed to understand some of the descriptions of planned activities, no matter how simply they were phrased. When she came to the unit, other than commenting that she had already been there to see the child psychiatrist, she made no spontaneous remarks or requests.

It was decided which age group Amber would join and also which class group. The teacher agreed to contact Amber's school to find out how she had been while in school as well as what work she had been doing. It was also agreed that Amber would start individual occupational therapy sessions, that there would be work with the foster parents to help them with their difficulties and concerns about caring for Amber, and that work would continue in preparing for the legal proceedings in relation to the care order.

3 Arriving at the unit

Note

The chapters relating to Amber's therapy are all written in the first person by the occupational therapist. The chapters begin with a description of the therapy sessions, followed by any teaching points arising from the session. The last part of each chapter discusses issues in clinical supervision.

AMBER'S FIRST DAY AT THE UNIT

Amber arrived as a day-patient on a Monday morning at 9.15 a.m. Her named nurse was there to greet her and introduce her to the group of children she would join. In the green group were the children and nursing staff she had met on her initial visit to the unit. The children in the group were all aged between 5 and 8 years of age. Later that day she would meet her teacher and go into class, and she would attend occupational therapy.

The group room is designed for children from the ages of 4 years up to 8 years and normally has up to 10 children in it, with a ratio of one staff member to two children. Within the unit there are three nursing groups, each one designed to match a developmental stage: one for the under 8s (green group), one for the 9 to 12 age range (red group) and a group for adolescents called blue group. The groups have these names because of the colour of the doors and most children recognize colours more quickly than complex names or numbers. Developmental needs can be taken into account by having the nursing groups divided in this way (Fig. 3.1), e.g. green group have smaller chairs than the adult chairs of the adolescent group; green group have lots of play materials while

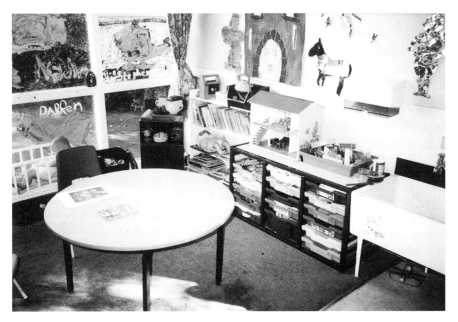

Fig. 3.1 The green group room.

the adolescent group has items appropriate for adolescent activities, such as music centres.

The teaching classes are also designed to meet the age range found in normal schools and teaching follows the National Curriculum. The class sizes are smaller than in a mainstream school and there is more time for individual work. Liaison with schools allows each child to follow the work-related topics found in their own school. The children spend about 3 hours per day in class. All the children receive occupational therapy twice a week. The three therapy rooms correspond with the nursing and teaching age bands, and are designed with the different developmental needs of each group in mind.

Meeting the occupational therapist

On the day that Amber arrived I saw her in the corridor and said hello to her and to her special nurse, who in turn repeated to Amber that I was someone whom she would be seeing later that day. Amber looked at me but said nothing. She moved slowly along the corridor into the group room holding her nurse's hand. She was reserved, unquestioningly accepting the day-to-day running of the unit and the routine of class and going to occupational therapy.

While in the group, she played some board games but quickly lost interest in them as she did not socialize with the other children. She looked around the group room and chose an activity that did not require her to interact with any children or staff members. This was how she spent the rest of the day: she responded to staff asking her to do things but the staff felt she was rather withdrawn and was not making relationships with anyone. Amber's isolation and her lack of interest in her surroundings was not the normal reaction of a child her age. She did not explore the room to see what was happening, or become involved with other children or staff. The size of the class is usually between two and five children, which meant that a lot of individual attention was given to each child; despite this, Amber seemed to be disengaged from her environment.

Later that day I walked into green group and greeted the various children who came to occupational therapy. In a day unit, it is impossible to hide the fact that you see different children. Many children find the idea of sharing you unbearable and are jealous of the therapy time that another group member will have with you. You often have to reassure those who are not coming with you that their turn is coming soon. Many children want to know what other children have done with you or seek out things others have made in order to destroy them. One child I worked with tied the door handle to the fire extinguisher as he left the therapy room, to prevent any other child from entering the room; such is the feeling of jealousy and envy that a child may have. A positive report from other children about their sessions is often of great assistance.

The first occupational therapy session

When it was time for Amber to have her first session, I said hello and explained who I was to her again. She had been told that I would be coming to see her and I assessed the situation to see if she was ready to come with me. She looked away from me at first then gave me a brief look as she made a movement towards the door. We walked along the corridor together then turned right and went outside, past the playing field and into the other building known as the activity unit (Fig. 3.2). The activity unit was where the occupational therapy rooms were. There was also a pottery room, a kitchen for the children to use, and a gymnasium in the same building (Fig. 3.3).

As we walked (Fig. 3.4), I explained that we were going to go to the activities unit and that the room with the red door was the room we were going to be in. As we entered the building Amber was able to see which room we were going to use. Once in the room I sat down and explained that I was an occupational therapist and that I knew from the child psychiatrist that Amber was living with her foster parents because something had happened to her that was not her fault. I said that I knew she had a sister and a brother who were living with her, and that she would be coming to see me so I could help her sort out her feelings. I said that what she was feeling may be because of different things that had happened to her. I told her that many children came to see me because they felt upset, cross or unhappy, or had other feelings, and that I tried to help them. I said that the way I tried to help was to allow her to play with anything in the room and to talk about the things that were important to her.

As I explained how often she would meet me, Amber looked around the room and asked many questions about her surroundings. 'What is this?' she said, touching a puppet, and 'What is that?' touching some sand. I sat next to the table as she explored the playroom. She continued to ask questions about the toys in the room and I reflected the feelings

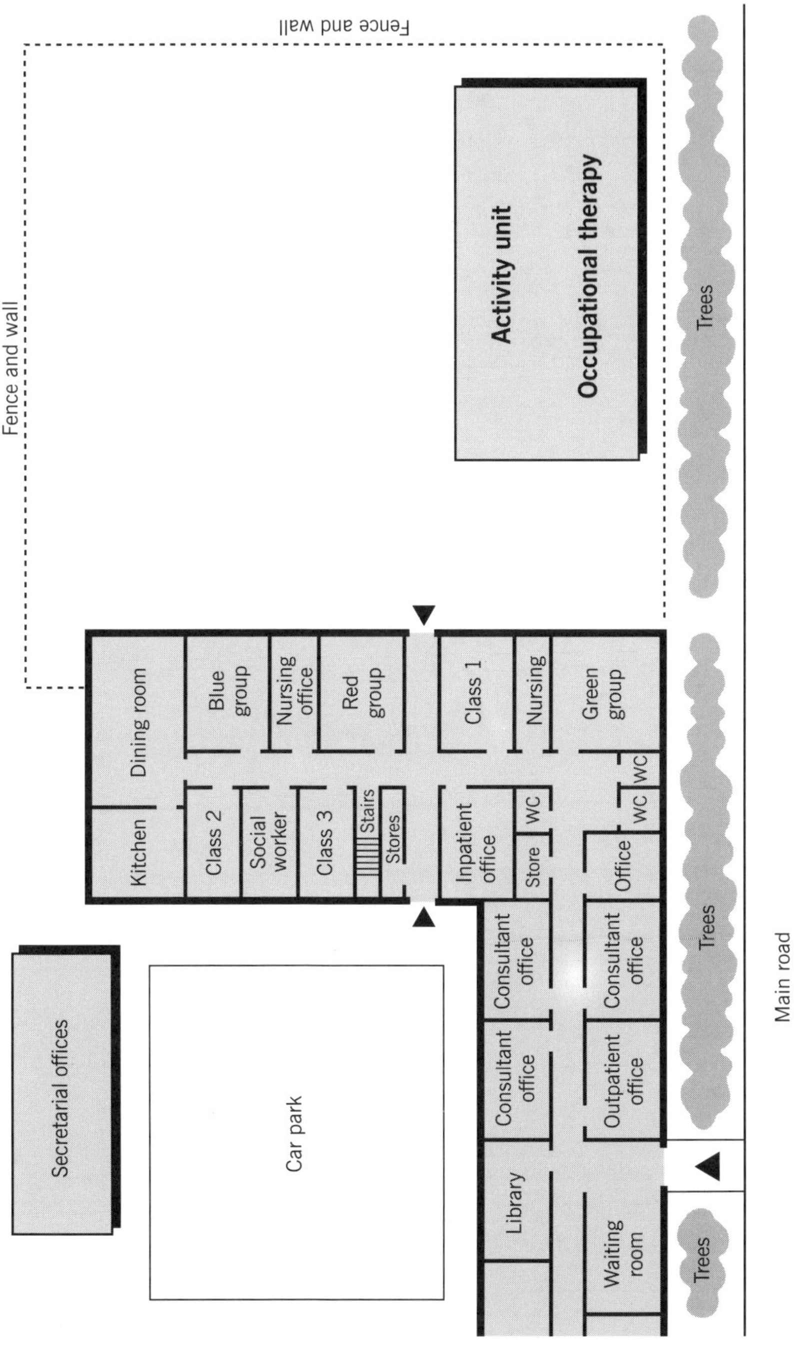

Fig. 3.2 The unit: floor plan.

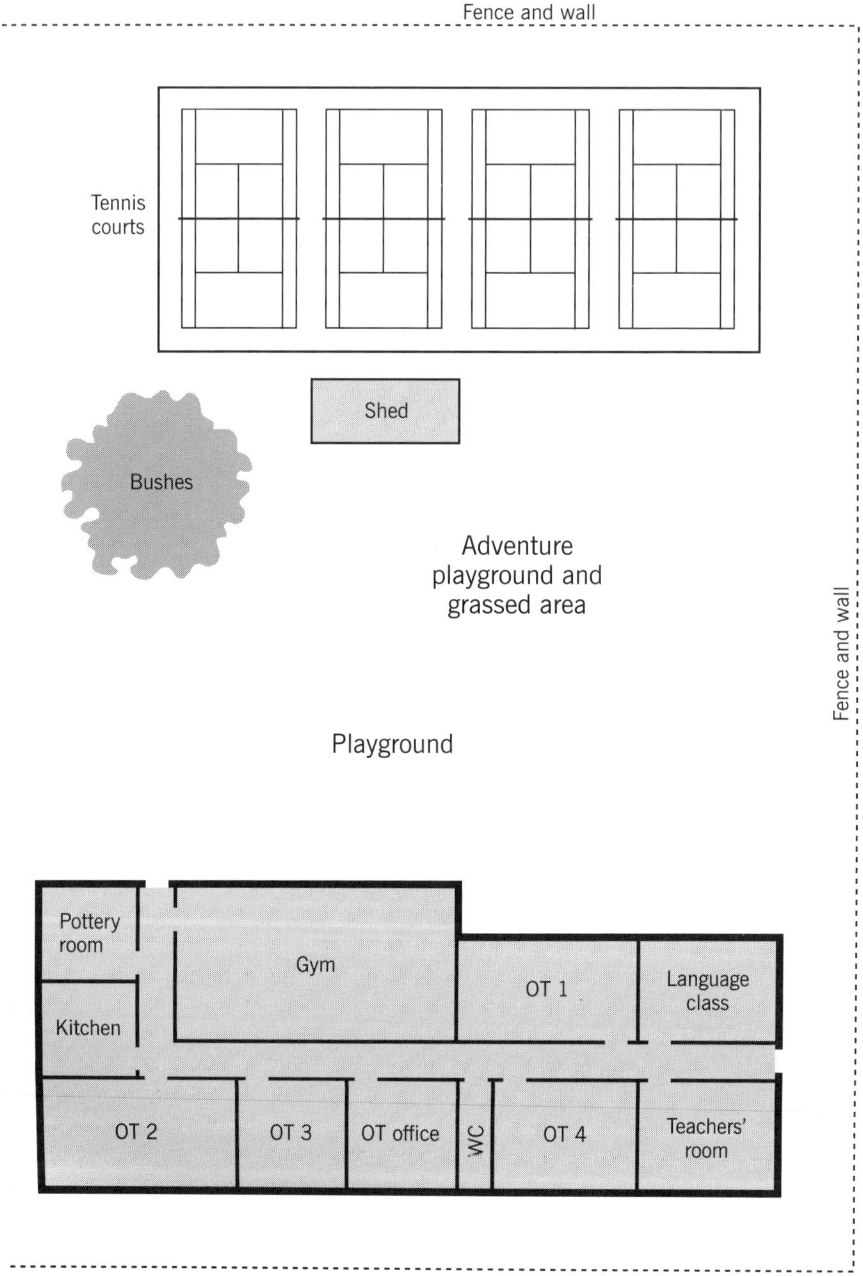

Fig. 3.3 The activity unit: floor plan.

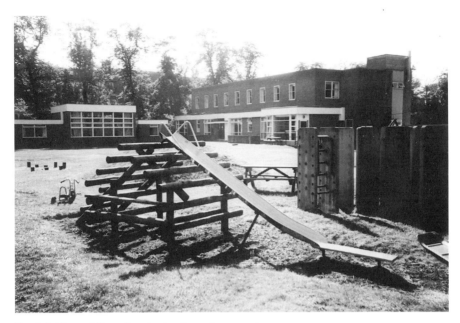

Fig. 3.4 The activity unit and adventure playground.

back to her by saying that it sounded to me as if she was not sure what things were and perhaps wanted me to tell her. She made no comment as she made her way around the room. She stopped by the doll's house and began to play with the figures, asking me if I would like to play with the doll's house with her. While she looked at the doll figures in the house she asked, 'Is this real?' about the objects that she touched. I repeated that she was asking if things were real but that they were toys and not real people or real chairs. She carried on asking if they were real over and over again.

After a few minutes Amber said, 'Do you know what Alan did?'

I replied, 'Yes, the child psychiatrist has told me that you have been hurt by Alan but that it was not your fault.'

'Do I have to tell you what he did?' she asked.

'Not if you don't want to.' I said. 'It's important to sort out your feelings after bad things have happened. I am not going to ask you questions. This is your time to play with the things you want to and talk about the things that are important to you.'

Amber carried on looking at the doll's house, standing next to it and picking up a toy TV.

'Have you any cards? Aunt Margaret has cards and she taught me a game.'

I said, 'Yes, I have some cards. It sounds as if you would like to play a game today.'

'Yes,' said Amber. 'Fish.'

I collected the cards from the shelf and Amber sat next to the table.

'How do you play "Fish"? I asked.

'You have six cards and ask the other person for say a six, she said. If they have some they give them to you. If they don't they say "Fish" and you pick up one.'

As we played the game, I realized we had 5 minutes left so I said, 'Amber we have 5 minutes left today before it is time to finish and go back to your group. I will see you on Wednesday at 10.00 a.m.' 'Will I see you again?' she asked. 'Yes in 2 sleeps time, on Wednesday,' I replied.

We carried on the game before I said, 'It's time to finish for today,' but Amber did not want to leave and began to play with my watch.

'What time does it say?' she asked.

'Quarter to 11, juice time. It's time to go today. I will see you again on Wednesday.'

Amber looked away from me and began to look back into the doll's house. I repeated that it was time to go and she looked up at me.

'Will I see you again?'

'Yes, I will see you 2 times each week, Monday and Wednesday.'

I stood up and walked towards the door. Amber followed and we walked over to the group room. Amber told me, 'It's juice time now. Look, I can see the other children in the group.'

The second occupational therapy session

On Wednesday I went towards the group room and found Amber sitting very close to her special nurse, looking slightly apprehensive.

'Hello, Amber. It is your turn to come and see me now.'

She looked at me and gave a faint hint of recognition.

'You remember Rick, don't you Amber ? I will be here when you get back,' her nurse said, encouragingly.

At this Amber left her side and walked with me to the playroom. Once inside she immediately went towards the doll's house and began to put it in the middle of the room.

'Are the dolls I played with still here?' she asked.

'Yes, they are in the doll's house,' I said.

Then she took out one of the dolls and hid it in a small doll's wardrobe with one door.

'Can you find it Rick?'

'You would like me to find the little doll that is hidden?'

'Yes,' she said.

This continued for the whole of the session; Amber would hide something and I would try to find it. I said perhaps she was trying to get me to guess about something that had happened or was hidden from me? She looked thoughtful and said, 'Yes.'

At the end of the session I said that there were 5 minutes left and Amber said that she did not want to go.

'I want to stay here forever,' she said.

'It sounds to me as if you enjoyed coming to see me if you would like to stay forever, but I will see you again on Monday. I shall think about you when you are not here and see you again next week.'

Amber took a little time to leave the playroom, saying again that she wished to stay but I reassured her that she would be coming back to see me and that I would think of her.

Reflection

Externalizing the concept of holding someone in your mind is an essential of therapy as the child will come to understand that she is thought about after she has gone. The therapist should also try to reflect the child's feelings back to the child as it shows that he has understood the child and allows clarification of what has been said. Reflection is a key technique in non-directive play therapy. It is an attempt to show the child that you not only understand what she *has* said but also understand what she is *trying* to say. Reflection can be carried out through repetition and putting into words the mood or feeling that the child is showing. It is an attempt to help the child link actions with true feelings and thereby gain insight into herself.

The game of hiding objects for the therapist to find is often initiated by children who are exploring what can be made explicit and brought into the open. The reflection used with Amber was acknowledging that she wanted the therapist to find the little doll over and over again. The therapist reflected that he thought she was trying to make him guess about something, to which she had replied, 'Yes.' Many children play in this way and it seems to serve as a vehicle both for building a relationship and for allowing things unsaid to be spoken about. The acknowledgement of sad, angry or hurtful feelings is not easy and takes time. The challenge is to follow the child at an appropriate level and to try to understand how this may relate to her experiences.

The importance of the first session

The first session with a child is one of the most important because it is the first opportunity to start to make a therapeutic relationship with the child. It is the relationship between the therapist and the child that underpins all that happens in therapy.

The therapist needs to be alert to the child's anxiety and to the fantasies she may have about why she is going with him. The therapist should explain what he knows and establish that he will devote all his time to that child during the session. In some circumstances, it is important for the therapist to ask the child why she thinks she is coming to see him; when it is appropriate to do this relies on clinical judgement and on being alert to the interaction in the room. The therapist should explain in clear, age-appropriate language what he is there for and what is going to happen. If a child seems not to go towards a plaything the therapist may have to suggest something for her to do; it is important to distinguish between a child who is assessing the situation, and weighing up what to do, and a child who is paralysed with fear.

The guiding principle of unconditional regard and acceptance of the child as an individual should always be present and the child should know that the therapist will communicate with her at a level which is appropriate and comprehensible to her, without intruding into her space either physically or emotionally.

For some children the fact that a session is ending is a shock and they wish to prolong it. A child who is worried about this needs to be reassured that she will be seen again. (The therapist reassured Amber in this way when he said she would see him again in 2 sleeps time. He did not know her cognitive level of functioning and was trying to reassure her that she would return.)

THE FIRST CLINICAL SUPERVISION MEETING

Later that day I met with the child psychiatrist for clinical supervision. Supervision is a vital aspect of child therapy; having undergraduate and postgraduate training is not enough. All those engaged in therapeutic work should be supervised to allow reflection and consideration of the therapy session, and to help the therapist to identify and understand the dynamics and relationship themes that emerge. Supervision is common in child psychiatry units and may be from someone of the same or a different discipline.

We discussed Amber's arrival and how the unit had been prepared for her and how she had been prepared for the unit. She had visited and met people on her own territory and at the unit. She had met her named nurse and she had been greeted by that nurse on her first day, providing a continuity of her care.

We felt that the use of non-directive play therapy was the best intervention for Amber at this time, together with milieu therapy provided by the unit. Milieu therapy is the use of all disciplines in providing a therapeutic environment for the child. All staff, from the domestic staff to the professor, are important in maintaining a therapeutic environment. The power of the environment to enhance change is considerable; the power to maximize accessibility to change comes with having individual therapy.

Non-directive play therapy

Non-directive play therapy developed from the humanistic school of psychology and is a way of allowing a child to get in touch with her feelings via play. Play is a child's work and is the vehicle for many developments, ranging from the development of hand eye coordination and cooperation with other children, to the working out of problems.

Many children will use play as a way to understand the world they live in. Play may be neutral, projective, destructive, social, constructive, age appropriate or regressed (i.e. below the chronological age).

The task of the therapist is to understand what the child is feeling and what the child is thinking, using play as the medium. The therapist accurately helps to reflect the child's feelings back to her to help her develop insight into herself. Non-directive play therapy was first described by Virginia Axline in her book *Play Therapy* (1989). It is a common method of treating children, providing an opportunity for a child to play out her feelings and problems. Her fears, anger, hatred and feelings of failure are played out in the therapy room. Some children require something more than an individual session once a week and so the unit provides 5-days-a-week attendance, where the effects of milieu therapy can be dramatic in changing perceptions or behaviours.

I told the child psychiatrist that I had seen Amber in a playroom designed for children under 8 years of age as, in my experience, children with similar backgrounds to hers often required a therapeutic environment which would allow any form of regression to occur. Regression often takes the form of emotional and motor behaviours usually seen in a child younger than the chronological age of that child. For example, a 7-year-old child may spend time with sand and water, pouring the sand, feeling it and enjoying the mess. Children of 7 do enjoy sand, especially on beaches, but at this age they are often building castles and use the sand for elaborate make-believe games. Feeling the sand, pouring water in and making a mess are more commonly seen in children who are 3 or 4 years of age.

Allowing a child to be in an environment in which to regress gives her psychological space (Fig. 3.5). The expectations in this environment are different from those in a classroom or in a family unit. It is important that in the therapy room there is time to think and to reflect.

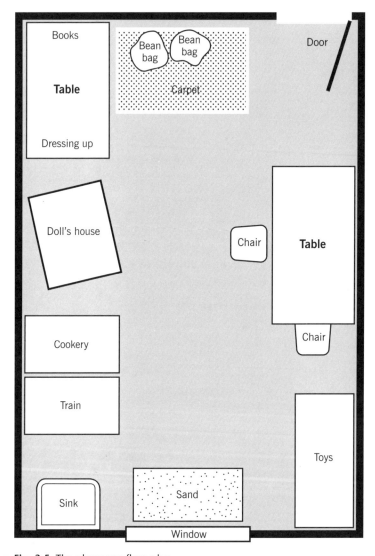

Fig. 3.5 The playroom: floor plan.

The playroom

The playroom is an important part of therapy. It must contain a number of play items that will be used by children of different chronological ages and different emotional ages (Fig. 3.6). It should have toys that allow

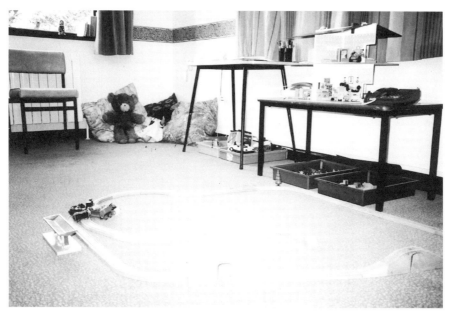

Fig. 3.6 A typical playroom.

expression, such as toy animals and materials for painting and drawing, and toys which may be used symbolically, such as telephones and a tea set. There should be access to a water supply, a sand pit, a small table and a chair. There should also be creative materials, paints and crayons and a soft beanbag to sit on. The toys which can be used in play therapy are:

- Neutral toys, e.g. jigsaws, table games and construction sets for various age groups.
- Regressive and/or aggressive toys, e.g. a nursing bottle, bubble-blowing equipment, sand trays (with wet and damp sand, and toys for sand play), sink and water, clay (non-firing), hammer toys, balsa wood and a few tools, finger paints and a large teddy bear.
- Toys for projective play, e.g. doll's house with furniture and doll's house people, transport toys (cars, fire engines, police cars, etc.), paper for drawing (with crayons, felt tips and paint), soldiers, wild and domestic toy animals, puppets, plasticine, equipment for making things (scissors, elastic bands, staplers, etc).

We then spoke about how important the concept of her time might become to Amber as it is unusual for a child to have time reserved for her twice a week with an adult who is interested only in the child. I had decided to see Amber at fixed times to allow her to understand when she would be seen. The other reason for this was connected with the therapeutic concept of 'holding', as described in the writings of Bion (1962). From a psychological viewpoint it was important that Amber knew at least one person was thinking about her and that there was a space for her which she could readily bring to mind. Most children can think about the familiarity of their home environment and know where everything is; they know that their parent(s) are thinking of them and that the parents know where they are. Amber needed this sense of security in her therapy sessions.

The child psychiatrist asked how the first session had gone. The first meeting and first session are vital when conducting therapy, as much of what follows builds on the success of the first meeting in establishing a relationship. The child must feel that the environment is helpful not frightening and should sense that she is coming to therapy for a purpose and that the therapist is there to help her. In the space of a few minutes a therapist has to judge how the child is feeling and act appropriately. You may have to bend down to the child's level or to stand back a little to allow some space for the child. Amber had looked a little apprehensive but also made a motion to move which told me that we should not delay but go. In talking with her as she walked towards the playroom, I felt I was building up a relationship with her. What is said in the first session is as important as what is done. A therapist needs to convey that he is aware of what has happened to the child, find out what the child *thinks* is going to happen, and set the therapeutic scene.

Amber moved swiftly into the room and began to explore it. Some children need more time or a little coaxing to explore the playroom. Amber asked if I knew what Alan had done, making it clear that there were things we both knew about. I explained briefly what I was there for and why she was there. I also tried to convey my interest in her being at the unit by my non-verbal communication, e.g. relaxed body posture, nodding my head in agreement, and a nonthreatening pose, and my interest in her feelings by not asking questions but by reflecting on the situation, e.g. that the first days in a new place were strange. The use of reflection is important because the aim is not to ask questions, or place one's own values upon the child, but to allow the child a space in which to sort out confusing events in her life. The therapist often uses the same words and phrases the child has used in order to convey an understanding of what the child means. The fact that many children have been involved in trauma of one type or another means that the pace of therapy needs to allow the child time in which to come to understand what she is feeling and why, especially as the child will transfer onto the therapist those feelings that she has had for her own parents. These feelings come from the child's conscious or subconscious and are often related to anger and rage.

Preconscious and conscious

The use of non-directive therapy is often regarded as the way for a child's preconscious to become conscious whereas psychotherapy is the way that the unconscious becomes conscious. Two of the most common forms of therapy are either client-centred therapy known as humanistic psychology, which tries to help an individual by reflecting his or her immediate feelings rather than by analysing them, or psychotherapy. Both therapies try to resolve emotional strife or upset by trying to find its causes. Non-directive play therapy relates to client-centred therapy and relies on helping a child to get in touch with feelings that are either conscious or lying just below the conscious level but not in the subconscious, i.e. in the preconscious. Psychotherapy aims to help a person become aware of his feelings by talking to a trained therapist who interprets those feelings, feelings which are often from the person's subconscious.

Amber had shown me by her play in the doll's house that certain things in her life were hidden and that she wondered if I could find out about these things, and perhaps give her some answers to these secret worries. The concept of time had proved to be very important to Amber as she had wanted to stay for longer and had found it difficult to understand that I would be returning at another time. The child who finds the concept of time difficult to grasp often has a poor sense of secure attachments from her original parent(s) so it is essential to have fixed times each week and to reassure her that she will return to see you. It is a unique experience for many children to spend time with an adult who is interested only in them. They soon realize that the adult will give them undivided attention, without interruptions, and will concentrate on trying to help them solve the problems they are experiencing.

Amber had been able to confide in me that Alan had done something, having first found out that I knew that what she had told the child psychiatrist did not have to be repeated. This may have allowed her to broach the topic of the abuse because she did not have to start from the beginning but could tell me what she wanted, knowing that I knew she had been abused.

We finished the session by concluding that the first two meetings had gone very well. Reports from the nursing group and teacher suggested that Amber was settling into the unit and starting to form, albeit very superficial, relationships with both staff and children. We felt that Amber was going to be able to make use of the therapeutic space that was being offered to her.

4

From play to pottery

Amber continued to attend occupational therapy twice a week, always on the same days and at the same time. She began to settle into the rhythm of the unit and there were hopeful signs that she was able to be less superficial in her interactions with others. She was beginning to develop strong relationships with both her named nurse, teacher and therapist. Although she could not follow the National Curriculum and had difficulty in forming peer relationships, we all felt that she was making progress.

GLUE DIAMONDS

As I arrived at the group room door I saw Amber sitting at one of the tables looking at a jigsaw on the table. I walked over and said hello and told her that it was her turn to come to the playroom. She looked at me quizzically but made a move to stand up. She came with me towards the door and accompanied me to the playroom. As we walked into the activities building she asked me what the sign on the first door said.

'That is the pottery room Amber. Children go into there if they want to make some pottery. Do you want to look inside?'

She shook her head and walked into the playroom ahead of me. As I went to sit down she began to look at the doll's house. She looked at the furniture, gently examining the small chairs and the table. She picked up the toilet and looked at it briefly before placing it back in the bathroom of the doll's house. Then she wandered around the room as if to explore it. As she walked towards the sand tray, she picked up a Russian doll from the windowsill and said that she knew what it was.

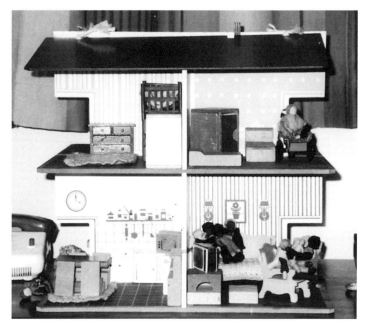

Fig. 4.1 The doll's house.

She sat down next to the table and began to open the doll. As she did this she asked me if I knew what was next.

'I think you want me to guess what will be next?'

She shook her head vigorously.

'What do *you* think is next?'

She did not answer but carried on undoing the doll until all the pieces were out on the table.

'How do you put it back – does this go in here?'

I nodded and said, 'Yes, sometimes it is hard to know how something goes back to what it was.'

She then chose another piece and asked if this was next; again I replied it was correct. Amber then moved away from the table and I said that it seemed hard to know what to do today. She looked at the beanbag and asked what was stuck on it. I replied that it was some glue that another child had spilled by mistake onto the bag. Amber began to pick at it and break off little pieces. I said she should be careful as the pieces may be sharp and I did not want her to be hurt. As I said this she looked up and asked if I would help her pick the glue off.

'They look like diamonds. Where can we keep them?'

'We could make a little box from cardboard and keep them in there if you want.'

She nodded and I picked up a piece of card to show Amber how to make a box. She did not want to cut out the shape with the scissors but readily offered to use the stapler after the shape was formed. As the little box was finished we placed the small pieces of glue in it. We had 5 minutes left as we finished putting the glue inside the box and I asked her what she would like to do with it. She replied that she wanted it left in the room. I placed it on a high shelf explaining that it would be safe there. Amber then began trying to tidy up saying we would finish soon. I acknowledged how difficult it was to end our time together and after a little while she left the playroom.

THE DOLL IN THE DUSTBIN

The next time I went to collect Amber she was with her named nurse and I was told that she had a cold. I said I was sorry to hear that she had a cold and wondered if she would still like to come with me to the playroom. Amber looked up and said, 'Yes, do you want me to go with you?' I said that I would like that. She smiled and we both set off from the group room. As we walked across to the activities unit, Amber said that she had not known it was her time and was I sure that it was her time? As we entered the room I said that it sounded as if she wasn't sure if I wanted to see her but I did. I said I would be seeing her 2 times a week and repeated the days and times. She asked if we could make some more diamonds. I said yes we could and would she like the box she made last time? Amber was thrilled that the box was still there.

'You kept it for me' she said.

'Yes, I put it on the shelf for you so that when you next wanted it that is where it would be. We can make some more diamonds by putting some glue onto a cloth and leaving it to dry. There is no more glue on the bean bag. Or we can use the scissors to cut up the bigger pieces of glue. Which one do you want to do, or do you want to do both?'

Amber decided to cut up the pieces and as I gave her the scissors she began to thrust them into the beanbag. As she did this I wondered out aloud if perhaps she was feeling angry or upset as sometimes children stabbed at things when they were feeling like that. I reminded her that it was all right to feel angry and we should think of a way for her to be angry without cutting the cushion. I gently leaned over and removed the scissors from her hand, saying that I thought she was cross but that I did not want her to hurt herself with the scissors so I would remove them. She did not resist and asked if she could put the new jewels in the box.

Amber then moved towards the doll's house and began to look at the figures in the house. She placed the little doll in the small cupboard.

'She's in the dustbin.'

'You're telling me that the small doll is in the dustbin?'

'Yes, she's been naughty.'

I said, 'The doll has been placed in the dustbin because she was naughty.'

I mentioned that it was not very nice to be placed in the dustbin.

Amber pulled the doll out and then pushed her back in the cupboard. A few minutes later she pulled the doll out and having found a little piece of cotton thread left in the doll's house she began to tie the doll up, her face a mixture of full concentration and revulsion. Once the doll was tied up Amber pushed it back into the cupboard.

'It seems to me that someone is angry with the doll, so much that they have tied it up and pushed it in the cupboard,' I said.

'Yes and it will have no food,' replied Amber.

Having done this, Amber then began to move around the room where she found a feeding bottle.

'What is the bottle for?'

'It is for children to use if they want. Would you like to use it?'

Amber stared at me with a look on her face that showed delight at the prospect of drinking from a feeding bottle as she nodded her head in acceptance.

'I will fill it with water or would you like to do it?'

Amber gestured that she would like to fill the bottle and she carefully began to unscrew the top then she filled it with water. She had a little difficulty putting the top back on and I helped her with this. As I gave her back the bottle she immediately put it to her mouth and began to drink in a slow manner, savouring each mouthful. There were about 11 minutes of the session left and Amber wandered to the bean bag and sat down with her bottle. 'Can you read me a story?' she asked.

'Of course. Which would you like?'

She picked a fairy story called *Cinderella* from the shelf. As I read she curled up in a small fetal position and sucked on the bottle, looking sometimes at the book and sometimes into my eyes.

'We have 5 minutes left today,' I said, and the session ended in a peaceful, warm way. Amber moved from the bean bag and asked me to keep the bottle for another time and we began to walk back towards the group room.

CINDERELLA IS GIVEN A PIGGY BACK

When I arrived in the group room for her next session Amber was nowhere to be seen. She was hiding behind the curtain. As she peeped out upon hearing my voice I pretended that I could not find her. When the giggles and sound of laughter came from behind the curtain I moved across to it. 'Boo!' she said, as she came out laughing.

Once in the playroom Amber began to play with the doll's house. She took the little doll and said that it was being put in the dustbin. She then said the doll had been naughty. I wondered about the doll being naughty and said that the doll may have been scared to have been put in the dustbin. Amber did not reply but began to say that she was tidying the doll's house. I said that some things were very difficult to talk about and I understood why she was tidying up the house. Amber did not reply but having finished her task looked around the room and found the feeding bottle. As she filled it up she asked if I would read the same story as last time. She sat on the beanbag, pulling it close to the chair that I was sitting on. I began to read the story as she drank from the bottle. As I finished the story, Amber put down the bottle and said that the mother in the story had been bad and that Cinderella was good. She then said that we could play *Cinderella* and that I should be the mother and she would be Cinderella.

'What should I do?' I asked.

Amber said that I should pretend to get ready for the ball and that I was to be cross. As she said this she suddenly changed her mind and said that *she* would be Cinderella and that I could be the magic fairy helping her go to the ball. Amber moved around the playroom and as she passed the dressing-up box she picked out a hat.

'Pretend I am crying and you come and see me,' she said.

I replied that I would be the fairy who came to see if Cinderella was all right, but when I got there she was crying.

'Yes, she is crying and the fairy has to say that she will help Cinderella.'

As Amber sat on the chair she pretended to cry. I said, 'Hello, Cinderella. I am the fairy and I have come to help you. What can I do?'

'I can't go to the ball, please help me to go.'

'Of course. What shall I do?'

'Get some mice and a pumpkin,' she replied, as if I should have known what to do.

I gestured to describe the magic mice and pumpkin and Cinderella pretended to climb aboard. It was nearly time to go and when I mentioned that there were 5 minutes left Amber sighed, 'Why does it always have to be 5 minutes?'

I said I thought that she sounded sad at only having a few minutes left and she nodded.

'Can I have a quick story?' she said, grabbing a book and the bottle at the same time as she leapt onto the beanbag.

'You may have as much of the story as we have time for,' I said.

When the time came to end, Amber showed no sign of moving but as I stood by the door she said, 'Will you carry me over?'

'I know you would like to be carried over but you are heavy so you can have a piggy back instead, if you want,' I said.

Hearing this Amber jumped off the beanbag onto my back and we went back to the group.

USING THE CLAY

The next time I called into green group Amber was hiding behind the curtains again and I played the game of 'I wonder where she is,' until, as she did last time, she jumped out from behind the curtain with a big 'Boo!' As we went towards the room, Amber asked if she could go into the pottery room. Once in the room I told Amber about which things could be made and what the potter's wheel was. I explained that there were some shapes to make dishes and there were also objects in the cupboard that she could use to give her ideas. She looked around the room and then said, 'My mum was an artist. I helped her make some bowls once. Can I make a cup?'

I reflected back by repeating to her that her mother was an artist and that she wanted to make an article like the one her mother had made. I explained that she could make a cup on the potter's wheel and that first we needed to bang the clay on the table to get rid of the air bubbles, as they cause the finished objects to explode in the kiln while it is being fired. I then told Amber that the cup would not be ready that day and showed her some newly made clay objects, some which had been fired once and were biscuit fired (terracotta) and finally some which had been glazed and fired again.

Amber took some clay out of the claybin and began. As I had instructed, she began to throw the wet clay onto the table. She smiled as she did this. She stopped to check for air bubbles inside the clay and asked if it was ready to throw on the wheel. It was so she placed the clay on the wheel and began to kick the potter's wheel causing the clay to move around. In order for a pot or cup to be fashioned this way, water needs to be poured over the potter's hands onto the clay to allow the hand to move over the clay and not hinder the creating of the pot by friction. I told Amber that I was going to pour the water over her hands and as I did so she began to make the pot. As the water reacted with the clay the residue poured over her hands. Amber slowly stopped kicking the potter's wheel and began to look at the mixture on her hands.

'Ugh, it looks like poo,' she said.

I agreed and she then started putting the mixture over my arm, smearing it onto my forearm in slow deliberate strokes.

'You're putting the clay on my arm; it doesn't feel very nice.' I said.

Amber said nothing but continued to smear the clay on my arm.

'Can I put it on your face?' she asked?

I replied that it was fine to smear it on my arm but not on my face. I then repeated that it felt awful and that sometimes children try to show me how awful some of the things that have happened to them are, and that I was trying to understand the feelings that Amber may have had. Amber turned and gave me a long, hard look and then resumed making her pot which became a vase rather than a cup, and then became a wet clay mess. We cleared up the mess from the wheel and in turn washed our hands and arms, finally removing the overalls we had worn. We returned to green group and I said goodbye. Amber waved goodbye.

Setting limits

A child's ability to form a relationship with others is based on her early life experiences. As Amber was starting to make relationships it suggested that her early life experiences were not too damaging. Her mother and significant others may have provided good enough mothering (as described by Winnicott (1986). The fact that she could not follow the National Curriculum was more a symptom of her having emotional conflict than a learning difficulty.

The use of non-directive play therapy includes limits when and where appropriate. Harm to the self or to others should never be permitted and breaking objects should be seen in this context. Smearing my arm did not bother me and allowed me to think about what Amber might be thinking or feeling; smearing my face *would* have bothered me. Limit setting is acceptable in non-directive therapy. By reflecting back the underlying feelings and not allowing harm to occur the child is anchored in reality.

A feeding bottle should be judged as a tool to help the child to regress if she wishes. She should not be chastized or belittled for using the bottle. Very early feelings are often allowed expression in the playroom.

It is important to allow the child a choice of what she wishes to do. There are times when an adult has to help, for example to turn on a stiff water tap; however, choice should be available. Telling a child of the various options also helps: for example, 'You can leave the top like that and water may leak out, but putting it on another way it will not.'

Children often create spontaneous role play situations in which they take on and play through characters from their own lives. Care must be taken that the therapist follows the child's agenda and seeks clarification from the child as to what should happen, rather than try and play with the child in a normal adult fashion.

There will always be debate about physical contact between therapist and child. Some children wish to hold your hand, some wish to snuggle close to you, some to jump onto your knee, and others to ask for piggy backs or to be carried places. In a child psychiatry day unit a lot of physical contact occurs. In this instance, I felt that Amber was emotionally regressed and that a piggy back was a reasonable request to make.

CLINICAL SUPERVISION

When I met with the child psychiatrist, we began by thinking about the last time we had met and what had been happening in the therapy room. There was a sense that Amber was making relationships and that these were meaningful to her. She was beginning to notice other areas of the unit, such as the pottery room, and to pass comment on them rather than remaining in her own world where no one thing seemed to connect with another. The session with the glue we thought could be taken several ways. She seemed unsure about what to do or think when she saw the dried glue, which could be something nasty, like dried semen, or something nice, like diamonds. The session had felt slightly disjointed and we both felt that perhaps Amber was having to think about many difficult things at once, without being able to relate them to one another or being able to deal with them sequentially at this stage.

At the next meeting, I had sensed that Amber was not sure if I cared for her. We wondered if she was testing if I really *did* want to see her and to help her. Some children who are familiar with rejection find it easier to handle if they reject the adults first, so suffering less than they would if they waited until the adults rejected them.

The session resumed at the point where Amber had left, despite a 2-day gap. This is a common procedure in therapy and gives credence to the room and therapist as containers for the child's feelings. The glue had upset Amber and she had shown anger and hatred when using scissors as a weapon. The feeling of anger in the session was felt by the therapist, as was the sense that there were things that Amber needed to explore.

Defence mechanisms

The therapist needs to be alert to the feelings which are coming from a child. It is vital that the therapist feels what the child feels in an attempt to understand the child. Often a child's actions do not match her feelings. For example, a child makes a cup in the pottery room but when it is placed in the kiln and fired it explodes. The child sees this and *says* that she does not mind having a broken pot but the therapist senses that her *real* feeling is one of anger or of disappointment. The therapist then talks about the fact that it is all right to feel angry or disappointed, in an attempt to allow the child to express her true feelings. Feelings of anger and rage are particularly difficult to express and people use many defence mechanisms in order not to express them. These defence mechanisms are normal but unconscious ways to avoid anxiety.

There were fleeting glimpses in Amber's play of the effects of abuse and of being hurt. Children often, as adults do, take some time to sort through things that have happened to them, or that they have seen, and this type of play is not unusual. Amber finding the feeding bottle is a common occurrence as a child may need to regress. This was clear in Amber's session because she was giving out signals that she wanted to be a little baby who needed to be fed and cared for. Regression can provide a way for children to regain their missed childhood as they can have a bottle, be told stories and given food.

Amber also asked for a story and then moved into a role play situation. Her meaning was immediately apparent when she said that the mother was bad and that Cinderella was good. The concepts of good and bad are understood by young children, as are the concepts of right and wrong, and often they wrestle with the consequences of applying this understanding to their own situation. Did Amber feel that she was wrong for having been abused and breaking up the family? Or was she trying to work out whose behaviour was right and whose behaviour was wrong? Amber needed to come to terms with the fact that the person she loved, her mother, had not looked after her in a loving way. In attempting to understand this she needed to be able to feel that she herself had not been the cause of the abuse and neglect. Amber, like many children, had to understand and accept the reality of her life, something that would not be easy given her age and the abuse she had suffered.

Adults can be wrong

Children struggle with the idea that adults can be wrong. How can a child understand abuse? Life teaches them that there is good and bad, right and wrong. Developmentally, children of this age are egocentric and see everything (good or bad) as depending on them so, logically, they work out that if they are abused it must be because of something they themselves have done. As they grow older, children develop a sense of morality and guilt and are able to reason that if something bad happens, it must be because they have been naughty and deserve punishment. The combination of egocentricity and a knowledge of guilt and punishment, makes a very uncomfortable and distressing mixture for abused children, unable to understand that it is not they who are wrong but the adults.

Amber's role play was hectic and there was no sense of direction to it. It suddenly ended as the session was about to end, making the time seem rushed and incomplete. Amber had then asked for a piggy back.

Children are often emotionally fragile following a therapy session because of the feelings that the session has reawoken. It is important to be alert to this and to act accordingly. In giving Amber a piggy back I was catering for her 'little girl' feelings and also responding to a degree of trust. Amber was willing to put trust in me, as her therapist, to carry her without dropping or harming her.

I went on to talk about the last session that I had with Amber. I explained that during this time Amber had started the session in the group room by playing 'Peek-a-Boo.' This could be an indication that she wanted me to make the effort to find her, or perhaps of a fear that I was going to go without her rather than wait.

Amber then changed her mind about going to the pottery room. It was there that she mentioned her mother and, following that, began to smear me with clay. The child psychiatrist and I spoke about how children often try to make you feel as they may have felt, and that the smearing was therapeutically useful because the situation had allowed her to express a feeling in a contained and safe way. The way she smeared me, and the nonverbal communication that I observed, suggested that she was expressing herself tentatively at first to see how I received it. Amber may have been trying to show me how invaded and dirty she had felt. The clay was referred to as 'poo.' This is not un-common with children but smearing the poo onto the arms of someone you know *is* uncommon. We both felt that Amber was working very hard on an emotional level to try to understand what had happened to her.

The child psychiatrist connected this experience to the difficulty that Amber was having in relation to staying continent; it seemed that she was particularly stressed at this time and her wetting had not reduced at all. Amber was also unsettled in class but seemed more trusting of her teacher. She had also started to talk more to her nurse about her daily life with her foster family and had mentioned that she missed her mother a lot. She had added that it was nice to see her grandparents but she wished they would be nice to her mother. We felt that she was starting to deal with her feelings and we were both pleased with her progress.

5

The butterfly children

AMBER THE JEWEL

On our way to the therapy session we went past the pottery room to the playroom. Amber began to look at the sand and made comments about the pieces of sand and how they shimmered in the light. 'They look like jewels,' she said. 'Look at the sparkle. Did you know that amber is a jewel as well? Mrs P. told me that. Look at the sand. Let's pretend that it is treasure and you and I are looking for it.' She stood close to the sand tray and motioned that I sit next to her.

'Look at the shining jewels. Aren't they beautiful?' she exclaimed.

'We're looking at the jewels and they *are* beautiful,' I said.

'Yes, jewels are beautiful and my name is a jewel.'

'I wonder if you are thinking that maybe you are beautiful?'

'Yes,' said Amber.

Amber began to move the sand in the sunlight, looking at the glistening specks of sand. The dry sand poured from her hand and fell into the sand tray. She buried one hand and pulled it out only to rebury it again.

'Shall we look for some treasure Rick?'

'Yes, let's do that.'

'Look,' she said. 'There is some there in the corner, real treasure. Do people think I am beautiful?'

'Yes,' I replied, 'some people do. Sometimes *we* think one thing and others think another. You are not sure if you are beautiful but others think that you are.'

Amber gave a thoughtful look before she said that she would like the diamonds that were in the box brought down to the sand tray. I stood up and reached onto the shelf to bring the box of glue-diamonds down. As I gave them to Amber, she emptied them into the sand tray and commented on all the jewels being in the sand. She remained by the sand tray for another 10 minutes, gently picking the sand up and letting it fall, enjoying the tactile experience.

'Let us pretend that we are magic,' she suddenly said. 'Look, I can make the door handle disappear.'

I reflected back that we were indeed magic *and* that we could make things disappear.

'Yes,' and she stood up and went towards the doll's house.

At the doll's house she began to pick up the same dolls as she had used in the previous sessions and started to hit the little doll.

'She has been naughty and she is being smacked. Naughty, naughty, naughty girl!' shouted Amber, and then she threw the doll onto the floor before turning around to find the feeding bottle. I asked if she wanted the bottle filled up or would she like to fill it up herself? She said that I should fill it up. As I gave her the bottle she sat on the beanbag, curled up in a fetal position and drank from the bottle. I said, 'Sometimes it is nice to curl up and drink.' She nodded her head. After a couple of minutes she sat up and said that she was magic and that she had made the door handle disappear. I wondered out loud, as it was nearing the end of the session, if she had made the handle disappear so she could stay in the room longer. She said, 'Your watch has disappeared as well.'

Amber lay on the beanbag and then said she would like a story read to her. I asked her which one and she said the same as last time. I began to read *Cinderella* to her as she lay looking up at me. As I showed her the pictures she gulped from the bottle. Shortly before the end of the story I said that there were 5 minutes left. Amber said that my watch had gone so that there was more time left. I commented that sometimes it was very hard to leave, but I would see her again and that I would think about her in between seeing her next time. She lay on the bag showing no sign of moving as I finished the story. All of a sudden she asked for a piggy back. I agreed and we left the room and went towards green group.

A CLAY FAMILY

The next time I saw Amber she walked passed the pottery room into the playroom and headed for the doll's house. She quickly picked up the dolls she had used before and began an imaginative game about a mother doll, a baby doll and a big sister. In the story the mother hit the big sister and hurt the baby. Amber talked as she played with the figures, explaining what was happening.

As Amber played I was able to reflect to her that the mother doll seemed cross with the two children and that she had hit the older one. I also said that the children may have been frightened and hurt by this, and that sometimes grown-ups are cruel to children and that it was wrong for people to hit children.

As the play finished Amber turned away towards the feeding bottle. As she did so she placed the mother doll in an upside-down position in the toy toilet bowl.

'Can you fill the bottle for me?' she asked.

Amber took the bottle and sat on the beanbag slowly drinking the water. As she sat on the beanbag she looked at me and said, 'We have some chrysalis in our class. Mrs Smith brought them in for the class to see. They will turn into butterflies soon. I wonder how pretty they will be? Can we go into the pottery room?'

As the room was free we moved into the pottery room and Amber began to get the clay from the claybin and throw it on the table to expel the air from the clay. Amber squeezed the clay as she held it and threw it down onto the table with great force. She laughed at the noise that it made as it hit the table top. Amber began to fashion a few crude shapes and as she did so she commented that they were a family.

'Look, here is the mother, here is the father, these are the children, this is the boy and this is the girl.'

As she finished the last shape she had before her four pieces of clay. There were no features to each person, they were just rough shapes of an elongated nature. Amber, having finished the last shape, rolled them all together and began squashing the mass on the table. As she did so she had a look of repulsion on her face. I stated that there had been a clay family and now there wasn't one, and that sometimes it is hard when a family breaks up. Amber made no response but carried on smearing the clay on the table top.

'Yuk,' she said. 'It's poo,' and she began smearing it over the table and close to me. I stated that the clay *was* like poo and it seemed all yukky and not very nice. Amber gave me a look that suggested that I was right and then she left the clay on the table and went over to the area where other children's work was drying or was waiting to be glazed. She picked up a few pieces. I said that there were 5 minutes left and that the thought of the poo may have made Amber feel strange and that it was all right to do something else. Amber seemed not to hear this and continued to look at the other pieces of work and not wash the clay from her hands. I mentioned that she would need to wash her hands before going back to group. After about 7 minutes, with me prompting, Amber went over to the sink and slowly washed her hands.

THE BUTTERFLY SPREADS HER WINGS

When I went to the group the next time Amber was again hiding behind the curtains. As in the past, I pretended to look for her as the giggles of laughter grew louder, then she suddenly jumped out from behind the curtains saying very loudly, 'Boo! Can we go to the pottery room?' We walked across to the pottery room and having quickly put an apron on Amber rushed to get some clay out and threw it on the potter's wheel. She seized the water jug and began to wet the clay as she started the wheel turning.

'Look, it's horrible,' she cried, as she smeared it over her arm. 'Shall I put it on you?'

'I think you want me to feel the same as you do when the clay is on your arm. Yes, you can place it on my arm,' I said.

Amber smeared the clay onto my arms asking me how it felt. I stated that it was horrible; she repeatedly asked me how it felt. This continued for about 15 minutes until we both had clay all over our arms. Amber then placed it onto her face and wanted to do the same to me. As in the past, I did not let her but said that it must feel horrible to have the clay all over her body.

Amber stopped the smearing and went to wash her hands and face, commenting that she wanted to go to the playroom. It took some time to remove the clay from our arms and several minutes later we entered the playroom. Amber immediately began to role play the game about me being the mother and her being the baby. There was also the sister who she named Jo Jo. Jo Jo had magic powers and this protected the baby. This was done very quickly before Amber announced that we were both butterfly children and we could fly. She began to 'fly' around the room saying that I should do the same.

'Look, there is a flower! Let us land on the flower.'

Amber told me that there were other butterfly children but they did not want to talk to us.

'We are pretty, nice butterflies flying around in the garden. Let us pretend that we are in a wonderland where everything is free and happy,' she said.

I thought out loud that this world seemed very different to the world in the pottery room. Amber did not reply but carried on talking about being a butterfly and how nice her wings were.

'Let us pretend we do not know the names of things,' she said, as she 'flew' about the playroom sniffing the air and looking at the various objects in the playroom.

'What's this?' she asked looking at a chair. 'I wonder what you do with it?'

I mentioned that I thought the butterfly was trying to sort out what was what in its world, and that the butterfly was seeing if things were really what they seemed to be. In the last few minutes of our time Amber flew around asking me to do the same.

'This is a wonderland,' she said, and she went out into the corridor towards her group room.

ROLLER SKATING AND MASKS

The next time that I saw Amber it was a very warm day and she asked if she could go roller skating. Many of the children had been roller skating during playtime and I saw no reason not to let her do this. Amber put on her boots, helmet and knee pads and very carefully stepped out onto the path and slowly moved towards the tennis court as this was an asphalt area, perfect for roller skating (Fig. 5.1). As she slowly skated she asked if she could hold onto my arm as she needed to steady herself because she was not very competent on the skates. There were a number of cries of 'Aaagh!' and 'Oooh!' as she slid on the skates. Amber asked me to protect her from falling and I said that I would and asked her what would be the best way to do this. She felt that holding onto my arm was the best way. As we moved towards the

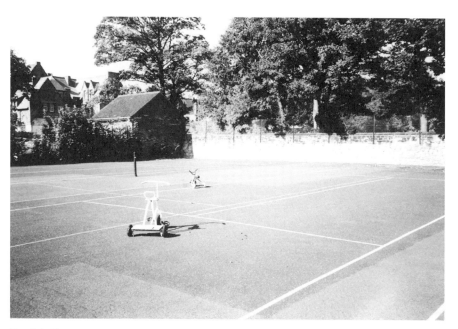

Fig. 5.1 The tennis court.

area Amber began to make up a game where I was in danger and she had to save me. This then became a game where *she* was in danger and I had to protect her, especially from falling. During the course of the game the fact that she skated and did appear to be falling added to my anxiety as to whether the play was real or not. The game went on for about 15 minutes and then Amber suggested going inside. As we walked towards the activity unit Amber asked if she could go into the pottery room and I agreed that we could. Amber went towards the plaster of Paris model making set that was also kept in the room. 'Can I make a mask?' she asked.

I asked her if she knew how to make the mask and she shook her head. Together we poured the plaster and mixed in the water and then poured it into the mask and allowed the plaster to set. Amber also saw a plastic mould of a bear and decided that she would also make this.

During the activity she asked a few questions about how the plaster set and why you had to mix it with water. As the models dried we cleared up and then with great delight Amber took the models out of their moulds and with a big smile asked if she could paint them. I offered her the choice of either the pottery room or the playroom in which to paint the models and she chose the pottery room. Amber took some time over which colour to paint them and carefully mixed the paints and applied them. She finished the last one just as our time finished. I quickly helped her make a box from card in which to take them back to her group room.

QUIET TIMES

The next time I went to collect her she was standing by the door waiting. 'Whose turn is it in OT?' she asked. I replied that it was her turn, that this was our usual time and would she like to come with me? She nodded her head and ran off down the corridor.

As we walked into the activities building Amber stood outside the door to the pottery room. I thought out loud that perhaps she would like to go into the pottery room? She nodded her head. Once in the room Amber ran over to the clay, quickly threw it onto the table and then threw it onto the potter's wheel. I helped her to centre the pot and she added the water.

Instead of trying to make a pot Amber began again to smear the clay over her arms and squelched it between her fingers, allowing it to drip out of her hands onto the wheel. I commented on the fact that it seemed to be not very nice and Amber said nothing but began to smear the clay onto my arms and then returned to squeezing the clay, listening to the noises it made while in her hands. Amber still said nothing, instead she became engrossed in the clay and the smearing.

I commented that sometimes we remembered things that were nice and sometimes we remembered things that were nasty. Amber remained silent, appearing to be lost in what she was doing with the clay. After a number of minutes she looked up at me and said that she wanted to go to the playroom. Sometimes a child will seem to be absorbed in an activity and not engage in dialogue. The therapist has to judge what may be happening within the child emotionally. The child does not have to be asked questions but should be allowed as much time as she needs as it is during these quiet times that a great deal of thought about the past may be occurring.

Once we had cleared up we went to the playroom where Amber asked for a story, filled up the feeding bottle, and curled up on the beanbag close to me. As I read the story I mentioned that there were 5 minutes left. Amber looked up and nodded as she drank from the bottle. As the time came to end we both stood up and walked back to the group room.

WHEN THE MAGIC DIDN'T WORK

During the next session Amber chose to be in the playroom. She walked in and immediately began to pick up the dolls which were in the doll's house.

'This one,' she said, pointing to the baby doll, 'is covered in poo and it's got snots all over it. The mother doesn't like it. Guess what she does Rick?'

I said the mother doll did not like the baby doll so much that she covered the baby in poo and snots and that Amber wanted me to guess what the mother doll did.

'Yes, guess what the mother did.'

I said that I could not guess as it seemed horrible what the mother had done to the little baby.

'She gave it some wee to drink! Her sister could not use the magic and the baby had to drink the wee!' shouted Amber.

I reflected that the magic was no use and the poor little baby had to drink wee and be covered in horrible things.

Amber held the dolls and pretended to give the baby doll a drink, and she made a crying noise as if the baby was crying.

'The baby is upset that it has to drink the wee and that its mother does not care for it,' I said.

Amber did not reply but threw the dolls into the doll's house and went over to the bottle and began to fill it from the tap. She put the teat on and began to drink from the bottle as she walked around the room before sitting on the beanbag. I said that sometimes things in a family were awful but not the children's fault, that grown-ups got cross and hurt children but the children were not to blame as they were only little. Amber asked for a story and curled up on the beanbag. She selected the story of *Cinderella* again and as we had 5 minutes left I told this to her. The time came to an end and we walked back to the group room.

The use of play figures in this imaginative way is often seen in younger children, as is Amber's running commentary on what was happening to the doll. Telling a story like this is a child's way of sorting out events in her own mind.

CLINICAL SUPERVISION

We met to discuss the work with Amber since our last supervision and I began by talking about the session that followed the last supervision. I explained that Amber had referred to jewels and linked this to beauty and her name. I had felt that Amber was perhaps trying to see herself as a positive person and I had asked her if she felt that people saw her as beautiful. We discussed the feelings that Amber may have had about herself and that she needed some concrete information that she was liked. She was making relationships with her named nurse and with her class teacher and from speaking to them it seemed that

Amber was beginning to work out if they liked her and, if so, why they did.

In the session she had asked for the diamonds that were still kept in the room. There had been a sense of relaxation as she allowed the sand to fall from her hands before she brought in the theme of magic. The magic seemed to be related to keeping the time in the playroom for herself and extending the time she had with the therapist. Amber had then shown me via the doll play some themes of a child being called naughty and being punished. These were very intense and were quickly followed by a regressed period where she was comforted by drinking from the bottle and having a story told to her. I did not reflect upon this to her because of the speed of her action and the sense that she needed to be able just to express something rather than have to think about it.

The child psychiatrist felt that the themes of beauty and goodness were in contrast to the doll play of naughtiness and badness, the power of which was so strong that Amber could not sustain the play and instead needed to have a source of comfort. We both felt that she was trying to sort out the elements of abuse and normality. Did people like her as a person? In the past, an important adult in her life, Alan, had liked her because she provided him with sexual gratification and had been an instrument for him to use and abuse. This is very different from most children's experience of adults who value them for who they are as a person. Amber needed to resolve why she had been abused and badly treated in the past if she was a normal little girl. We both thought that I needed to help her with the struggle with her identity as a normal little girl.

I explained how the session had ended with the request for a piggy back and how this seemed to relate to the little girl feelings and regression at the end of the session. Within therapy the issue of physical contact is one which has to be handled sensitively. Children can spontaneously touch your arm, perhaps when putting a plaster on you, or they may ask to sit on your lap for a story. Sometimes children will ask to be carried or to have a piggy back. Physical contact should not be denied but the therapist must be alert to what the contact may mean to the child and to ways in which the request may be allowed while keeping within the boundaries. For example, if a child asks to sit on your lap you can acknowledge the request but say the child can sit next to you. For more physical contact, as in a piggy back, you can allow this if it seen by others, i.e. by opening the playroom door prior to the child climbing onto your back and moving off into the public space straightaway.

I explained that the next sessions were linked together. Doll play and abuse had reappeared and had been expanded to include a mother figure. The figures had been formed in clay and included a father figure but these were quickly squashed up. In between the play there was a sense that Amber was able to start bringing aspects of the real world together, as when she told me about the chrysalis in the classroom. The child psychiatrist commented that this also seemed related to beauty and to a sense of change. The image of change from a powerless chrysalis to a beautiful butterfly was not lost on either of us. The sense that Amber was changing as she thought about her past was also evident when she made a plaster mask and bear shape. This was the first constructive activity that she had done. It was also age appropriate making both of us feel that she was moving towards her chronological age developmentally.

This making of concrete things, the mask and the bear, had been mixed with play involving smearing and explicit abusive episodes. The more explicit themes of abuse were later mentioned culminating in the last session where the baby had to drink urine. There were brief themes of magic and of protection, as when Amber played on the roller skates and needed to be protected and when the sister, Jo Jo, had magic. We both agreed that the nature of the play and the themes were consistent with a child attempting to sort out her feelings following a trauma. The relationship that had developed allowed an element of trust to be included. This trust allowed Amber to begin to bring some forms of abuse out into the open and to check out the therapist's feelings towards the abuse. There was a gradual exposure of more and more intrusive feelings involving faeces and mucous, while she also showed signs of normal development. In these sessions Amber was being more spontaneous and free, in comparison to her earlier sessions which were disjointed. However, therapy is often difficult in the initial phase as a relationship is built up and the child begins to learn that the therapist is there for her and that the time is hers. Reports from the other professionals also suggested an improvement in Amber and I looked forward to hearing about these at the next review.

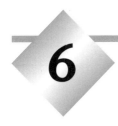

6

The legal framework and case conference

This chapter is divided into two parts. Firstly a discussion of the legal framework within which Amber was managed and secondly a description of the case conference for Amber.

THE LEGAL FRAMEWORK

Amber was the subject of professional concern so statutory processes were used to try to ensure her safety and meet her needs.

There was a high level of concern about Amber as she had made allegations of sexual abuse. There were physical signs consistent with this and, as well as the physical abuse, her mother was using drugs regularly and had a lifestyle which exposed Amber and her siblings to risk. There were worries about Amber's physical growth and development, and psychiatric examination had shown her to be a deprived and damaged child.

In the United Kingdom there is legislation to protect children, the Children Act 1989 (England and Wales). The basic provisions of the Act are to establish the following:

- The welfare of children is paramount.
- Children are best cared for by their parents wherever possible.
- A checklist of factors is to be considered which includes the wishes of the child as well as the child's cultural, racial and linguistic background.
- The state and the courts should intervene only where improvements will be made for the child.
- The concept of 'parental responsibility' replaces that of 'parental rights.'

- Local authorities have a duty to safeguard and promote the welfare of children in need and must also provide services for children and families.

At the time of Amber's initial referral she and her siblings had been placed in foster care by the local authority. This had been done against the wishes of Katherine, her mother, by the granting of an order by a court. The social services department had made an application setting out their reasons for concern and, having heard the mother's refutation of this, the judge had granted an interim order, and asked for a full assessment to be ready for a final hearing.

The child psychiatrist was asked to prepare a report for the court, providing an assessment of Amber's needs and making recommendations for her future care and management. This work was done on an outpatient basis and also in parallel with the work of other disciplines working with Amber in the day-patient unit. One of the principles guiding the assessment is to approach the situation with an 'open mind', in other words, it is not assumed that the child either has or has not been abused. The starting point is that most children will be cared for best by their parents. The child psychiatrist, therefore, interviewed the children, the parent and other members of the family who had a significant involvement in the child's life, observed interactions between members of the family, and carried out a family assessment. All documentation relating to the case was considered and there were formal discussions with other professionals involved from the educational, health, social work and legal professions.

A report was then prepared, taking into account the likelihood that the children had experienced or were at risk of experiencing significant harm, the needs of the children, and the capacity of Amber's mother to provide appropriate care for the children. It is important to consider in these situations whether any form of intervention would help the parent to improve his or her capacity to exercise parental responsibility, for example, by therapeutic work support. The conclusion reached was that Katherine was sadly not able to provide good enough care and protection for her children and that they should be placed in the care of the local authority with a view to placement in another family. The child psychiatrist suggested a detailed assessment of Amber's grandparents as possible carers for her.

This recommendation was accepted following a lengthy court hearing. The social services department then held a number of meetings and a reduction in the contact between Amber and her mother was organized. Contact between Amber and her brother and sister was maintained, but it was decided that the children should not be placed together in one family. Jenny and Craig were to be kept together and placed with a middle-aged couple whose own children had grown up and left home. This was a temporary arrangement but it was thought that it would be better to have clearer idea of Amber' strengths and difficulties before placing her permanently. In addition, there was little information about Amber's grandparents and their capacity to care for her needed to be evaluated. The work in the child psychiatry department was crucial to this assessment.

In separate criminal proceedings, Alan had been tried and convicted of a Schedule I offence (offences against children are categorized under Schedule 1). Amber had completed a video recording in which she was interviewed by a woman police officer about the allegations she had made against Alan. A social worker is always present during these interviews to act as a support to the child.

A memorandum of good practice is followed when using video inter-views. The videos may be admitted as evidence in court and may be sufficient for the court's needs, but children may also be called to give evidence in person. To do this a video link between the child, who is in a room away from the court, and the judge, jury and legal repre-sentatives, may be used. Alternatively, the child may give evidence from the witness box but a screen is used so that the child does not see the alleged perpetrator or vice versa. In Amber's case she was not called to give evidence but Alan was still convicted.

With regard to parental responsibility, Amber's situation was changed by the granting of a care order to the local authority. Whereas Katherine had previously been the only person who could act for Amber, for example, in terms of giving consent, this was transferred to the local authority, although obviously the mother's support was desirable and would be sought as long as she was in contact with her daughter. Amber's own wishes and feelings were an essential part of any discussions and were considered very carefully before any major decisions were made.

The work with children in Amber's position often begins after the court has made decisions about their care. Once Amber had been placed in short-term foster care regular care team meetings were convened to consider plans made for her care. Her progress in the child psychiatry unit was vital in considering her ability to cope with changes in care arrangements, the kinds of educational provision that should be made for her, and the frequency and nature of contact that she should have with her siblings and other members of her extended family such as her grandparents. A careful consideration of her grandparents' ability to care for and protect Amber was needed. Their difficult relationship with Katherine and their relative lack of involvement with Amber in the past had to be evaluated in detail.

CASE DISCUSSION

It is normal practice to review the management of a case on a regular basis with all the professionals involved. In England and Wales, this is done on a statutory basis when children are placed on the child protection register and also when they are in the care of the local authority as a result of a care order. The meetings are convened and chaired by independent chairmen for the social services department. The aims of the meetings are to receive and to discuss information concerning the child and her family, and to review work which has been done before planning the way forward. The meetings are usually attended by all those providing care for the child, those who have parental responsibility, and representatives from the education, health and social services.

The meeting for Amber was held at the end of March in the library of the child psychiatry department (Fig. 6.1). It was a cold and blustery day and the coffee was welcomed by everyone attending: the chairman,

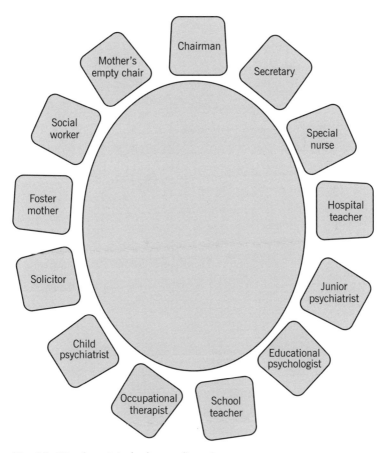

Fig. 6.1 Attendees at Amber's case discussion.

at the head of the table, Amber's foster mother; the secretary taking minutes; Amber's named (or 'special') nurse; her teacher; the junior psychiatrist from the child psychiatry unit; Amber's teacher from her local authority school; the educational psychologist; Amber's occupational therapist; the consultant child psychiatrist; the local authority solicitor and the social worker. An empty chair was left for Katherine, who had written to say she would be attending but who did not arrive.

The social worker

The chairman opened the meeting by welcoming everyone and explaining the purpose of the review. Information was given by the local authority social worker first. She reminded everyone that Amber had been placed on an interim care order at the last court hearing. She reported that Amber had remained with her foster parents who had found her behaviour troubling and difficult to manage at times. She also explained that Amber, together with her brother and sister, had some contact with her mother every 2 weeks. The social worker said that she took Amber out for lunch on an infrequent basis and had listened to anything she wished to tell her. On the last of these meetings Amber had been very tearful but on previous conversations she had lacked any emotion.

The foster mother

Amber's foster mother reported that Amber was usually quiet and helpful but to an extreme that the foster mother found abnormal and unsettling. Amber also seemed to have great difficulty remembering simple instructions such as to dress or fetch something from the kitchen. She also needed frequent prompting to get ready in time for outings but was generally washed and dressed ready for breakfast on unit days. She told the meeting that Amber was not interested in playing outside with other children and often seemed lost in thought and inaccessible when everyone was watching TV or playing a board game. The foster mother said that others, including herself, found this very irritating at times. She said that Amber ate well but was often troubled by nightmares and wet her bed on most nights. The foster mother quietly cleared this up and never made a fuss about it. Amber had recently started stripping her own bed and putting the sheets in the washing machine. The foster mother said that Amber masturbated on a daily basis but more often did this in her own room now and did not usually behave inappropriately when with others. She still needed to be watched but could be distracted if she started masturbating. Amber had never behaved in any other inappropriate way as far as the foster mother was aware.

The named nurse

The team from the child psychiatry department gave their reports next. Amber's named nurse reported that Amber had taken several weeks to settle into the unit. At first, she had stayed close to her special nurse and been very reluctant to leave her side. In spite of this, Amber had been very guarded when talking to her nurse and only in the last few weeks had she been able to hint that she did not like Alan because he did nasty things. Amber had also recently begun to engage in the various activities available and preferred to play in the Wendy house and with soft toys in a manner more often seen in younger children. When a child had fallen in the unit 2 weeks before Amber had become very angry because she thought the fall had been caused by another child. She had shouted at her named nurse about how wicked this was and said that the injured child had not been properly cared for when hurt. She went on to talk of how people should not be allowed to hurt children and when her special nurse agreed with her about this, Amber had said that sometimes bad things happened to children because they were naughty. She had listened to the nurse's response, which was to agree that children were sometimes naughty but that it was wrong for very bad and hurtful things to happen to them when they were naughty. The nurse had said it was better to help children to understand *why* they should not be naughty or rather not do certain things, but Amber did not make any further comment.

Amber had frequently needed reassurance that she would see her mother and grandparents but seemed unable to hold any timescale in her head, which meant she became distressed if she believed that she had missed a visit to any of them. Amber had not really made any friends in the unit and other children found her periods of abstraction very strange and annoying. There had been some attempts to make fun of her but Amber seemed unaffected by any of this.

The unit teacher

Amber's teacher in the unit said that her ability to concentrate was extremely variable and she had great difficulty writing anything on paper. Amber was a little more productive using the computer and parts of her work indicated that she might have greater ability than had been apparent at first. Amber found it difficult to sit down and pay attention on some days, and the fact that she was taught with only two other children allowed the teacher some capacity to accommodate this. However, the teacher felt that Amber would benefit from individual lessons and noted that she had responded well to work done on growing and caring for plants. Amber had successfully grown some peas and was planning to plant some lupins next month. The times when Amber sat silently and apparently uncomprehendingly in class were usually after contact with her mother. She had said that she felt very sad on one of these occasions when her teacher had sat and talked with her, and had said that she worried about her mother who was so beautiful and clever. She had said that she would like to be like her mother but knew she could never be that wonderful. This theme had also come up when Amber had made some mistakes in her mathematics, when she had torn up her book and said she knew she was hopeless and no good. The teacher had talked this through with Amber, taking a cognitive approach, but had not had a direct response from the little girl.

The junior child psychiatrist

The junior child psychiatrist said that in his sessions Amber was polite and answered practical questions, such as what she had eaten and what she done over the weekends, in a matter-of-fact way. He said that he did not feel that he had any significant relationship with her but that she accepted his regular checks on how she was progressing. He said that Amber still had some symptoms, such as flashbacks and symptoms of panic, but that these had decreased in frequency. He confirmed that Amber had grown a little in height and weight and that she had no urinary tract problems to account for the wetting. He also reported that Amber had had an EEG and neurological examination and no organic cause had been found for her periods of inattention.

The occupational therapist

Amber's occupational therapist reported that Amber had taken some time to develop a relationship with him but that he felt that this had now been established. The basic themes which had emerged related to who cared about and for Amber; the differences and conflicts between good and bad; the need for protection from bad things and how even magical protection sometimes did not work. He reported that Amber's sense of self-esteem had been very low but that more recently there were signs of this changing, in that she could imagine beautiful nice places and had also introduced the idea of things transforming, for example, a chrysalis into a butterfly. Her behaviour had included destruction and defiling, such as smearing, as well as an increase in her creativity shown by making a mask and bear from plaster of Paris.

The consultant child psychiatrist

The consultant child psychiatrist commented on the remarkable amount of progress Amber had made in the last 9 months and how, although they struggled with Amber at times, the foster family clearly had succeeded in providing a sound base of care for her. In addition, it seemed that Amber was benefiting from her time in the department of child psychiatry where she had input from so many professionals and was able to use what they had to offer.

The solicitor

The chairman said that it was unfortunate that Katherine had not been able to attend as she obviously could have provided a considerable amount of information that would have been of great use to the meeting. The solicitor acting for the local authority pointed out that the final court hearing at which the local authority would seek a care order would take place in 3 weeks time. It was expected that this would be opposed by Amber's mother and evidence would be called from the child psychiatrist. The child psychiatrist had submitted her report at the request of the social services department and she had supported their application for Amber to be removed from the care of her mother. The solicitor added that Amber's grandparents had made an application for a residence order, which was opposed by Katherine and there was a high level of acrimony between the parties.

The school teacher

Amber's school teacher said that she had not had any contact with Amber for some time, apart from having visited her briefly in the child psychiatry unit immediately before the meeting. She commented that Amber had remembered her and had shown her the plant she had grown and talked enthusiastically about her work on the computer. The teacher commented that Amber seemed to have grown in height and also seemed less anxious than the last time she had seen her.

The educational psychologist

The educational psychologist said that he did not know Amber personally but, as it would be his responsibility to organize education for her when she left the unit, he needed some idea as to whether she would need special educational provision. He pointed out that Amber had not been succeeding at school and there was a high level of concern that she was not as able as other children in mainstream education. Amber's teacher in the child psychiatry unit said that she was not sure what Amber's actual ability was, but at times there were indications that she may be more able than was originally thought.

Amber's nurse was sure Amber was of average intelligence at least but that her life experiences were handicapping her ability to relate to the formal demands of the classroom. The child psychiatrist thought it may be better to wait a little longer before completing an assessment to determine Amber's educational provision. This was agreed and the educational psychologist said he would see her for this purpose at an agreed time.

The meeting ends

The plan agreed was that Amber would continue to reside with her foster parents, have regular contact with her mother and grandparents, and continue to attend the child psychiatry department 5 days per week. A date for the meeting to reconvene in 3 months was set and the chairman thanked everyone for attending. The nurse asked who would tell Amber about the meeting and it was agreed that Amber's foster mother and social worker would do this, and staff at the child psychiatry unit would also be ready to answer any of her questions.

SUMMARY

Amber presented in several settings as a child who seemed disconnected with the world around her, being described as preoccupied, absent-minded and lost in thought. In addition, she seemed to find it very difficult to form any emotional contact with people and they found this, in combination with her lack of motivation and inability to respond to instruction, very frustrating. We saw this behaviour as a response to the huge changes she had had to cope with in the recent past in terms of separation from her mother and home, in the context of the abuse she had suffered, and in her inability to trust anyone as a result of her impaired care and attachment in early life. Her nightmares and wetting were symptoms not uncommonly seen in children who have been abused. The masturbation was frequent and initially without any sense of a need for privacy, and this, too, is a behaviour encountered in abused children.

Amber presented as a child with an extremely low sense of self-esteem and poor self-confidence. These are often characteristics of children who have not developed a sense of being valued and who have not been given a sense of their own importance as individuals. It must also be remembered that a child in Amber's situation could be experiencing flash-backs, when the traumatic experiences are relived briefly, sometimes in response to a trigger in daily life, such as a colour seen or a phrase spoken by someone. Amber also had an idealized view of her mother and a great need to be with her but this warm attachment had not been returned by Katherine, and had become an unrealistic, unattainable and much-wanted fantasy in Amber's mind.

Amber also presented as a child whose cognitive ability was questioned. This is often seen in children whose minds are so full of the bad experiences they have had that there is little room for the ordinary demands of the classroom, or even some aspects of daily life. As these children also have a very poor sense of self-esteem it can be difficult to help them to engage with others and start to move along an appropriate developmental path.

THE MULTIDISCIPLINARY TEAM

The work with Amber had been done by many members of a multi-disciplinary team, in a situation where Amber was safely and consistently cared for by her foster parents. Work by a team can be difficult and there is a great need to preserve team cohesion and cooperation. Each discipline had a great deal to offer to Amber and an important role to play in engaging her emotionally, socially and cognitively. It was important for each member of the team to be clear what his or her main task would be and how this would fit in with the work of the team as a whole. Planning and coordination needed to be flexible and constantly discussed, hence the need for regular team meetings and a frank exchange of views in a constructive format. One of the characteristics of working with children like Amber is a high potential for splitting within the team, with team members taking opposite views about decisions based on their own unconscious feelings. For example, a team member may say that a child needs to be rescued from a situation through adoption when the best solution for the child may be rehabilitation with her parents. Or a team member may want to ascribe blame for a child's challenging behaviour rather than working out why the challenging behaviour is occurring.

The ability of professionals both inside and outside the unit to work together is often a key to the success of the intervention and provides a safe, consistent and cohesive caring environment in which the damaged child can start to recover and return to the business of normal growth and development.

7

Holidays and cinder toffee

INTO THE KITCHEN

Amber was waiting by the group room door when I next went to collect her. She smiled and asked if it was her turn. Upon hearing the affirmative she raced off towards the playroom. As we walked past the kitchen she said that it smelt nice; I asked her if she would like to go into the kitchen and she nodded. As we walked in, I explained that children could make different things here and I wondered if Amber knew what she would like to make? She nodded her head and said, 'Cinder toffee.' I explained that cinder toffee was a hard thing to make because it required sugar, butter and golden syrup to be boiled together and that we could make it but she had to have some help because it was dangerous. I went on to explain that in the kitchen there were rules about safety because there was an electric cooker and I did not want her to get hurt.

Amber asked what was in the cupboards and I explained where the various utensils were and in which cupboard the ingredients were kept. Amber looked into the wall cupboard and spying the raisins said, 'I like raisins.' I acknowledged what she had said and took a paper baking case from the cupboard and said that Amber could have some ingredients in this. She chose some raisins and some glacé cherries. While Amber ate the food I found the pan and the scales and placed them on the bench top, explaining to her what the various pieces were. 'Can I have some margarine to eat?' she asked, and I replied that she could not as it may upset her tummy but she could have some more raisins. Accepting this Amber ate quickly and looked around the room enquiring what the various objects were. There was the extractor fan, the fire blanket and other objects found in a therapeutic kitchen.

As Amber weighed out the sugar and margarine I told her that I was going to go on holiday next week and that I would see her once more this week and then not for 2 weeks. She asked if she would see another occupational therapist and I replied that that would not happen because it was difficult for another person to get to know her in a short time. I mentioned some of green group who had been on holiday and come back.

'My special nurse has not been on holiday, she won't go,' Amber said.

I reflected that sometimes we got cross when people went away and maybe it did not seem fair to her that I was going away. I said that she might be angry if I went away because we saw each other twice a week and now there was going to be a break. I reassured her that it was all right to have these feelings.

Amber said nothing but squashed the sugar and margarine together very hard with the spoon. As the ingredients were to be cooked on the hot plate I asked Amber to sit by the bench and asked her if she would like to put some margarine on the baking tin to help stop the toffee from sticking to it. I also asked if she would like to look at some recipe books. As she did both she began to ask more questions about the room.

'What is this for?' while looking at the fire extinguisher.

The toffee was almost complete and we placed it in the refrigerator to set as we began to make a bag to keep it in. Amber asked for some more food and I said that it was almost lunchtime and I understood that she wanted lots of food but she could only have some raisins. Amber grunted and looked cross but accepted the raisins. With the washing-up done and the toffee in the bag we set off back to the green group room.

GOING ON HOLIDAY

The next time I went to collect Amber from the group room she was playing a game with another child. I stood in the room and mentioned that it was her turn for OT and asked if she would she like to finish the game that she was playing. She said nothing but carried on with the game. The little boy with whom she was playing said, 'Can I come instead of Amber?'.

I said I could understand that he wanted to come instead but I would see him at his usual time; this was Amber's time and she was deciding what to do. I crouched by the pair of them when Amber suddenly got up and said, 'Are you coming or what?'.

Amber went into the playroom and began a quick game with the dolls, hitting the little doll and saying it was naughty and its mum would not look after it. I said that it was very difficult knowing that I was going on holiday and that Amber might be feeling very cross. Amber said nothing but threw down the doll and asked. 'Can I go into the kitchen?'.

Once inside the kitchen, Amber climbed onto the bench and started to look inside the cupboards, pulling out various ingredients and saying that they were her favourite foods. I asked what she wanted to cook but she ignored me and began to eat some raisins. I placed a paper bun case in front of her and said that she could fill the bun case with food rather than place her hands in the jars. Amber ate the food quickly and then looked at my pen which was placed in my top shirt pocket. 'My mum had a fountain pen. Can I make some cinder toffee?' she asked.

As we selected the ingredients I commented on the fact that Amber was thinking about the pen her mother used to have and I wondered if Amber was thinking about other things from the past. I said perhaps my holiday made her think that I was leaving her and that this might make her feel cross. Amber listened but said nothing. However, as she mixed the sugar and butter together she said, 'Why are you going on holiday?' I explained that I was coming back and I would see her again. I told her that in the 2 weeks when we would not see each other we could think about each other and sometimes this helped when you did not see a person you liked. Amber carried on mixing the cinder toffee and asked for some more food, adding 'and a drink.'

I reflected that she would like some more food but added that because it was lunchtime she could not have any. I then asked if she would like a drink of orange juice instead of raisins. I poured some orange juice into a cup and gave it to her. The activity was nearly over and, as I placed the cinder toffee into the refrigerator to set, I helped Amber to make a bag and mentioned that there were 5 minutes of the session left. I then repeated the fact that I would see her in 2 weeks time. The bag took the same time to make as the toffee took to set and we both placed the toffee in the bag, having first removed it from the refrigerator. Amber managed to break a little off and eat it as we did this. We left the session on time and walked back towards the group room.

The next time I went to collect Amber I had been back at the unit for 1 day. As I walked into the group room Amber did not look up but continued to play a game with her named nurse. I stood beside her and asked if she would like to come to occupational therapy. She said nothing. I waited for a little while and said that I had been away and that she might have been cross with me but I had come back as I said I would. I repeated my offer for her to come with me. 'I don't want to come with you,' Amber said. I explained to her that this was acceptable and that it was her time. I would go to the playroom and wait there in her time in case she changed her mind. I left the group room and went to the playroom.

Just 3 minutes later I heard Amber 's named nurse saying, 'Which room do you see Rick in?'. I opened the door and said hello to Amber and thanked the nurse for bringing her. Amber walked into the playroom with her head down and went towards the doll's house. She picked up the small doll and began to move it around the house commenting that it was looking for its mum. I reflected that the little doll was looking for its mum and wondered how it felt if it could not find its mother.

'Sad,' replied Amber. 'She can't find her mother because she is naughty, and the mother does not want to see her.'

I said that the small doll felt sad because she had been naughty and that the mother did not want to see the doll because of this. Amber nodded and said, 'Can we go outside?'. I said that because it had started to rain we could not. 'You don't want me to play anywhere,' she said.

I talked to Amber about feeling let down and left alone because I had gone on holiday, and said that it was fine to be cross. I said that perhaps she felt like the little doll because she had been left by her mother. I also said that I had gone on holiday, because people go on holiday not because of anything Amber had done.

'Can I have a story?' she asked. I asked her which one and as I went to pick it up she filled the feeding bottle and settled down on the beanbag awaiting the story. We finished the session after two stories. Amber asked for some extra time because she had missed a little and I explained that it was her choice. I said I knew she had been cross but there was still the same amount of time. She reluctantly finished.

MAKING A CAKE FROM SAND

The next time I went to collect Amber, she was by the door and she asked whose turn it was for OT. I explained that it was her turn and repeated the day and time that I saw her. Amber raced across to the playroom with me quickly following. As I walked into the room Amber had already begun to play with the doll's house. The scene she enacted showed the mother doll being cross with the baby and not giving it any food. The mother then changed her mind and locked the doll in the cupboard. 'She is in there because she naughty,' said Amber. As I reflected that the mother seemed cross with the baby and that the baby had been placed in the cupboard, Amber walked across to the sand.

Amber sat next to the sand tray and began to look at the sand, letting it fall from her hands. 'Can I put some water in the sand? I'm going to make a sand castle,' she said. As she placed some water into the sand she stirred it around commenting that she was making a cake. She stirred the mixture adding some paint from nearby. I wondered out loud if the cake was a good cake or a bad cake. 'A bad one,' she replied. Amber became engrossed in the sand, mixing the water, sand and paint into a viscous mess. She made a few half shapes using the sand castle moulds but quickly destroyed them. 'The cake is for the baby. She's been very naughty.' I said that I wondered what the baby had done to have such horrible food. Amber did not reply; instead she continued to mix the sand, swirling it about in the tray. The time was coming towards the end and I said that there were 5 minutes left. 'Will you keep the sand like this for me until I come next time?' she asked. I replied that I understood that she wanted the sand to be the same for next time but I could not keep it the same. I could draw a picture of how it looked, or we could put some of the sand into a bucket and save it until next time. Amber agreed to the last suggestion.

We spent the next few minutes putting the mixture into the bucket and then into the cupboard. 'Will it be safe ?' she asked. 'Yes,' I replied. Amber and I left the playroom and returned to her group room.

GLOOP AND MAGIC

Amber was waiting by the door the next time that I went to collect her. She was full of enthusiasm and began telling me what she had been doing in the group room as we walked across to the playroom. Once inside the room Amber went to the cupboard and began to take out the sand mess and deposited it in the sand tray. She began to mix the mess with the fresh sand and called it gloop. 'Look at this gloop I've made. It's some food.' I said that the gloop was food and that she wanted me to look at it.

'Let's pretend that I am called Lesley and I have some magic, and that you are the baby and you have a sister called Jo Jo.' Amber set the scene and a quick storyline emerged in which Lesley gave the baby some of the bad food and made it drink urine. The sister Jo Jo tried to help by using some magic but it would not work. I thought that this was very sad for the baby, who was only little, and that Jo Jo was brave to try to use the magic to make Lesley not harm the baby. Amber quickly lost the story and asked instead for a story to be read to her. She chose a story and sat on the beanbag while I read to her. After a period of time we left and returned to the group room.

GREEN TILES AND WHITE TILES

The next time that we met was a few days after the anniversary of Amber arriving at the unit. She had succumbed to a heavy cold and had had a few days off. She had been sick and required a lot of physical attention from the nursing staff as she had a variety of cuts and minor ailments, such as a sore throat. She had also developed some cold sores and was being treated for those. As I walked into the group room, Amber was seated at a table looking very ill. I approached and she looked up at me with a half smile. 'It's your turn for OT,' I said.

She rose slowly from her seat and began to walk towards the playroom. Once in the room she began a game in which the tiled floor was the site of some disgusting mess. The green tiles were snot and the white tiles were the ones that we were allowed to walk on. Amber insisted that we walk around the room trying to avoid the snot covered tiles. This lasted about 4 minutes and then Amber seemed to run out of steam and flopped onto the beanbag. She complained that her throat was sore and that she felt hot. I asked her what she would like to do, adding that I thought it might be best to go to the sick room and lie down until she could go home. Amber thought for a little and then said she would like to do that. We walked towards the nursing group and soon Amber was being looked after by her named nurse.

Attendance at a session

There will be times when child may not wish to attend a session and this should always be taken seriously. The best course of action is to acknowledge the situation and state that the time is available to the child, as you first stated in your initial meeting with her. You should return to the room and await her. It helps to have something to do while waiting in case she does not come. If the child is reluctant to come with you on your first meeting ask if anyone can come with her, for example, a parent. Once the child accompanies you with a parent or another person, allow a period of time to reflect on her feelings and ask if the other adult can leave. There may be a gradual phasing out, with the adult sitting near the door, then the adult going outside the door, and finally the adult waiting in the designated area. Children will often try to extend their time with you or ask for extra time. It is always better to keep to the exact amount of time. Sometimes if a session is shortened, for whatever reason, I will explain to a child that we can add the missed time onto another session. In the example, I reflected the feelings and the fact that there was no more time. It is not a time to bargain with the child and is fair to everyone because, if you make different rules for different children, they may meet and find out, with the obvious result that some children will be jealous, upset or angry because they do not get extra time.

Children may wish to keep the room the same or have the arrangement of toys the same for the next time that they attend. There are various ways of doing this, such as drawing a plan, taking a Polaroid picture, or working out a compromise whereby some things are kept unchanged and others altered.

CLINICAL SUPERVISION

Later that day I met with the child psychiatrist and discussed the sessions so far. I started by explaining what had happened since we last met. Amber had discovered the kitchen and had made some sweets. There had been a sense of the therapist feeding her in the session and of her demanding sweet, nice foods. The feeding had occurred in the context of explaining that the therapist would be going on holiday. Amber wondered, almost casually, who she would see instead, before affirming that her named nurse would never leave her, even for a holiday. She seemed able to accept the fact that a separation may have an emotional effect on her, that she may be cross. The session was about feeding. There was a sense that some good food was being kept from her, as had actually happened when she had wanted some more and was offered raisins because it was lunchtime. The child psychiatrist asked if she had seemed sad or cross, explaining that if she had been more cross then this could be seen as a more normal reaction. I had replied that she seemed more cross than sad. We both saw the ability to engage in an activity and to plan and follow instructions as a continued sign of her progress.

The next time I returned I had been met with a rebuff: if I was going to leave her then she would leave me. It was short-lived and Amber went to the playroom accompanied by her named nurse. She may have been checking to see if I had kept my word and was waiting for her in 'her time period.' We both felt that the use of doll play was Amber's way of trying to work through some of the things that had happened to her. The child psychiatrist speculated that the doll play might also have been Amber's way of trying to see if she was really bad and if being bad was what was making the therapist leave her. This theme was impossible to explore in the playroom but Amber allowed more exploration of what going away might mean to her once she reached the kitchen. She made reference to the pen, which was similar to her mother's, and asked why I was going on holiday. The child psychiatrist thought that this was also linked to the fact that Amber's mother went away and did not return. She wondered if Amber felt abandoned by the therapist and if the break in therapy represented a threat to their

relationship. Amber might have been worried that if the therapist returned, the relationship might have been altered and he might not
want to see her. The pen was a link object and Amber was able to make
use of the reflection to ask me why I was going on holiday.

The theme of eating was still prevalent, with Amber wanting to eat
lots of food in a quick, rushed manner. Although a limit was applied and
contained by the use of a bun case filled with raisins, Amber still asked
for more food. The therapist explained that this would spoil her appetite
and asked if she would compromise with a drink of orange juice.
The session ended with the making of the bag and the placing of the
toffee into the bag, with Amber eating some of the toffee. The child
psychiatrist asked why I had not said anything and I replied that the
actions of finishing the session were conducted in a warm but brief
manner, with a good deal of eye contact, and that when Amber ate the
toffee I had felt this was a way of saying the relationship will continue
and making sure there was a pleasant end before the next time we met.

The session following a holiday is clearly an important one for therapy.
After my holiday, Amber was faced with the reality that people *can* be
trusted to return, as well as her own feelings of anger and hurt.
She decided to reject me and I accepted her feelings and I went to the
playroom to wait for her.

The child psychiatrist thought the play with the doll's house and the
talk of being let down were probably Amber's true feelings and wondered
if there could have been another way of dealing with the situation.
Amber probably felt that even the weather, with the advent of rain, was
against her doing what she wanted and maybe I could have commented
on that when I was talking to her. The child psychiatrist suggested
that perhaps I had been apologizing rather than trying to make explicit
my understanding of Amber. In hindsight, I could have been more
thoughtful with her.

The next time, Amber returned to the theme of the neglected baby and introduced the concept of bad food. I commented that bad food was a common theme in therapy and the child psychiatrist agreed. We discussed the use of good and bad food to represent all the good and bad parts of parenting. The fact that Amber wished to keep the sand/food for the next session indicated the importance of this activity to her.

The theme of the bad mother also recurred but again was lost and proved too difficult to develop. The child psychiatrist noted that Amber's cold sores and general ill health coincided with the anniversary of her being removed from her mother's care. We both pondered on the psychological effects that this was having on Amber, and the child psychiatrist said that Amber was having a difficult time in group, where she was confrontational and angry with both her peers and the staff. She was also impulsive and seemed oblivious to dangerous situations. She was wetting a lot and it seemed that nothing was going right for her. In class, where there was a clear structure, she was more at ease, perhaps because she did not have to focus on her feelings as much as she had to in therapy sessions.

8

Snots and sycamores

COLLECTING SEEDS

'Can we go out today?' asked Amber.

It was now September and the trees were just beginning to lose their leaves.

'Yes,' I said, 'but we have to put our coats and gloves on if it is too cold.'

Amber wanted to walk around the unit, not in the areas that she knew but towards the main buildings where the sycamore trees were. As we walked towards them, Amber told me that we were going to collect some things and take them back to the playroom. She told me that she had been to this part of the grounds with her class and that they had looked at the trees and talked about autumn. I said to Amber I wondered if she was thinking about the way things change and how they change.

'Yes,' she said. 'All the leaves fall off the trees and then it becomes winter and it's very cold.'

'Yes,' I said, 'it is cold in winter. It is nice to be wrapped up warm.'

We arrived at the trees and Amber asked me to help collect the seeds that had fallen onto the ground and put them in my pocket. They were sycamore seeds and we scooped them up until my pockets were full. We then walked back to the playroom where Amber asked that I empty my pockets and said that we should start to sort them out. The sorting out took the form of throwing them in the air and giving points or a score for how good they were at flying.

'Let's throw them in the air and see how good they are. We can give them marks. We can give them marks like very good and good,' said Amber.

The categories that Amber chose were very, very good; very good; good; not too good and bad. We sat on the chairs with the sycamore seeds placed upon the table and she threw one into the air. As it fell towards the ground it spun in the helicopter fashion that characterizes sycamore seeds.

'What sort was that one? I know it was a good one,' said Amber.

We gave it the category of good and the seeds began to pile up into groups. While we were doing this Amber was talking about which were the best ones and which were the worst.

'What is this one? I bet it is the worst. No, it's a very good one,' she said.

I commented that she seemed to be trying to sort out the good and the bad parts of the seeds and that perhaps it was like having to sort out the good and bad parts of her life.

Amber asked, 'Do you think that I am good Rick?'

While she threw the seeds in the air I replied that I did think she was good and that sometimes children worried if they thought that they were not good but that she had not done anything wrong.

By this time there were 5 minutes left and I asked what Amber wanted to do with the seeds. She said we should keep them so we needed to write out the categories and store the piles for, perhaps, another day. The seeds that were not used were placed in a plastic container and I placed them all on the high shelf of the playroom.

BAD SEEDS

The next time that I collected Amber from the group room she was standing by the door.

'Who have you come to see?' she asked.

'You, it is your turn for OT,' I said.

She smiled and ran off ahead of me towards the playroom. I ran after her and as I walked into the playroom I saw that Amber had pulled the chair towards the bottom of the shelf and was about to step onto the chair to reach up for the sycamore seeds.

'Shall I get them for you'? I asked.

She nodded and I moved the chair back to the table, handing her the plastic box at the same time. Amber sat on the mat and began to lay out the categories and select the seeds from the box. The game then took on a new meaning whereby the bad seeds were squeezed and the green part of the seed was called a snot. This snot was a very bad thing and had to be placed in the plastic container.

'This is a dustbin. Let's put the snot in the dustbin,' said Amber.

A lid was put on the dustbin and Amber then hit the dustbin very hard, shouting that she was getting rid of the bad things.

'Bad, bad, bad, go away, go away!' she called.

Amber never said what the bad things were. She did not need to. She placed the green seed/snot in the plastic box and beat it with her hands. As she did so she had a very determined look on her face.

'Rick, I have been getting rid of the bad. It won't come again.'

'Yes, you have got rid of the bad and it will not come again,' I replied.

'We have 5 minutes left before we need to return to the group.'

Amber looked at me and said, 'Yes, 5 minutes left. Can I stay a little longer?'

'You want to stay longer but it will soon be time to finish. I shall think about you and I shall see you again on Monday.'

A TRIP IN THE CAR

The next Monday, Amber walked into the playroom and began to pick up the teddy and the doll.

'Let's pretend that these are our children and that we are going on a journey to see the doctor. We have to stop Alan from hurting them. Do you know what he did?'

I replied that it seemed important to protect the children from something Alan had done but I did not know what it was.

'He put his finger up their bums, you know.'

I said what he had done was wrong and that the children may have felt scared or hurt.

'Let's take them to the doctor,' said Amber.

'Which doctor are we taking them to?' I asked.

'Dr Anderson, she will see them. Come on, Rick. Get in the car.'

As she said this, she began to move the two chairs together and place the beanbag behind them so that they looked like a car. Amber then proceeded to direct a role play where I was, at different times, a driver, the father of the children, and Dr Anderson. The children were lifted towards me by Amber and they whispered to me what had happened. I reconfirmed that it had not been their fault and that Alan was wrong to have done this.

'They are only little,' said Amber.

Amber then told me to get into the car and said,

'I will drive. Are the kids all right? Let's go to Africa.'

We drove along in an imaginary way for a few minutes, then Amber said,

'Let's go to the police and tell them what has happened to the children. There're only little you know. He was 54 not a 2-year-old.'

'Yes, he was older and should not have done the things he did because he knew what he was doing, he was not little.'

Amber stopped the car and we were at the police station.

'You tell them what he did,' she said.
I asked whom I should tell.

'The policeman,' said Amber.

I moved into the role of the policeman and than back to being myself, telling myself that the children had been hurt by Alan.

'What shall we do Amber?' I asked.
'Let's arrest him,' she replied.

I then said we could pretend that the cushion was Alan and she nodded in agreement.

'Come on you. Off to the police station.'

As I did this Amber laughed in a very nervous way.

'What shall I do now Amber?'

She seemed to be lost for words so I said that I would put him in the cell.

'He has a key you know, Rick.'

'Alan would not have a key if he was in a prison cell. He would be by himself and not have a lot to eat. He would not be allowed out unless the police allowed him and then they would be with him.'

At this point I began to tell Amber that the police arrest people when they think they have done something wrong. Then they are sent to prison when the judge says they have to be punished for doing something wrong. The prison would not be a nice place because people did not like grown-ups hurting a little child the way that Alan had hurt her. Amber seemed to listen to what I said and then said,

'Let's take the kids to the beach.'

I replied that we could go to the beach in our game and that there were 5 minutes left. In these 5 minutes we drove to the beach and Amber and I pretended to have a picnic with the children. We quickly packed the chairs into their place and tidied up the room. As we were about to leave Amber chose to go and look at the sand.

'It's time to go today, I said. 'I will see you again on Wednesday.'

Amber looked up at me and said, 'Yes, I will see you on Wednesday.'

She then began to walk towards the door and ran off, with me following, towards her group.

FEELING PROTECTED

Wednesday came and Amber was standing at the door of green group. 'Who have you come for?' she asked. I said that it was her time now and wondered if she would like to come with me to the playroom. She smiled and raced off towards the door with me running after her. Once inside the room, Amber asked for the treasure box containing the pieces of glue, the 'diamonds.' As she placed them on the palm of her hand she said,

'I like you, Rick. I love you. You protect me from my mum.'

I said that she had a number of feelings for me and that one of these was a feeling that I helped her to be protected from her mum. I spoke of people liking others and I wondered if her mum had done anything that might have hurt her.

'She used to throw tapes at me,' Amber said, solemnly.

'That must have been scary for a little girl. Did it hurt as well?'

She did not reply. Instead she placed the glue pieces back into the box and rushed over to the sink and grabbed the feeding bottle. She began to fill the bottle and told me that we were going to play a game where she was a little baby and I was the mother. There was also another girl who was the sister. Amber crawled onto the beanbag and asked me to place a piece of material from the dressing-up box over her. I did this and waited for my next instructions.

'Let us pretend that you are cross with the sister.'

I asked for clarification and followed my orders, telling the imaginary sister off, telling her as Amber told me, that she was a bad girl. Amber lay on the beanbag and said that I should tell the sister off. She then said that I should find a rope and tie her up and she would be the baby watching from the cot. I said that the sister must have felt very scared to be tied up and that it did not seem a nice thing to happen to a little child. Amber said nothing and drank from the bottle. It was 5 minutes before we were to finish and Amber asked for a quick story. She paid little attention to it and soon it was time to go.

THE POWER OF MAGIC

The next time we went to the playroom Amber began to play with the wet sand. She asked me to pour in more water and then said that there was enough. I sat near the sand tray as she squeezed the sand between her fingers. As she began to experience this tactile sensation she began to spread the sand up onto her arm. She turned to me and spread some onto my arm. I thought out aloud that Amber had covered her arm in sand and now she was doing the same to me.

'It's yuk sand', she said. 'It's all yukky and horrible.'

'The sand is all yukky and you are spreading it over me and yourself. We are both feeling the yukky sand,' I replied.

She carried on pouring the sand from between her fingers into the sand tray, pushing her hands into the sand, burying them and rediscovering them. Amber suddenly stood up and washed the sand from her hands at the sink. Amber said that she would like to play the same game as the other day and said that I should be the mother and she would be the baby, then she said that the sister was magic and the magic could provide food. Amber did not direct the session but concentrated on showing me what the sister could do.

'Look, there is some food. Look the plate is broken. No it's not, it is fixed with magic.'

I said that it was good that the sister had magic and could fix things and get food for the baby and mother. She continued telling me about the magic, that the sister had asked me to show her a toy plate, or toy cup, and telling me that it was broken, before saying that the magic had fixed it. Amber then said that she was a little baby and she was 1 month old. Her name was Lesley and I was her mum. I repeated this back to Amber and she replied,

'Yes, and you are going to put me to bed in 5 minutes.'

As she said this, she climbed onto the beanbag and began to make baby noises. She then asked for the bottle and some baby food. I reflected that she was the baby and that the mother had to feed the baby. As I gave her the bottle Amber said,

'Count the bubbles Rick.'

I began counting the bubbles as she drank from the bottle. I said to her that we had 5 minutes left and she told me off for not counting the bubbles. I apologized and said that it was difficult to end sessions, and that counting bubbles was fun but it did not mean that the session was finished. At the end of the session Amber became magic.

'I'm magic but you don't know. I can fly, I can take you by the hand but you don't know. I'll make some wings for you.'

Amber motioned some wings onto my back via her magic and then with a wave of her hand made them work. With this gesture we 'flew' out of the playroom.

Therapeutic space

The use of other areas apart from the playroom is often debated by therapists. Should you keep therapy in the playroom and so maintain the theories of containment and holding, or can a child also use a space out of the therapy room? Some children need space out of the therapy room either for developmental reasons or because the therapy room space has become too intense. Working in a developmental framework allows a child to pass from activities using gross motor skills to activities using fine motor skills; working in different areas allows the development of play from parallel to sharing, and from imaginative through to constructive play.

Therapy should also begin from where the child wishes it to start. In two consecutive sessions Amber decided she would continue working with the seeds. Many children are able to pick up from where they finished at the end of the previous session, despite a week's break separating the sessions. This lends credence to the concepts of therapeutic space and the holding of the child in the therapist's mind. Many children in weekly therapy say 'remember yesterday' about something when, in fact, there has been a break of a week since they last saw the therapist.

Role play

When the therapist is asked to role play he must be careful to notice the effect of the role play on the child. Often, much of the meaning of the role play is based in fact and this can upset a child. When asked to be angry with a doll or imaginary child the therapist should never shout but use a different voice and should check with the child if that is what she wants to happen. Sometimes it is useful to stop and comment on what is happening, for example, to say 'that must be horrible' or 'that must make you feel very sad.'

CLINICAL SUPERVISION

We began by discussing the fact that Amber had been out of the therapy room and the possible reasons for this. She did not need the time for exploratory play but showed her need to bring something to the session, in this case the sycamore seeds. The seeds were linked with thoughts of change and how the seasons changed. We knew that Amber was changing and that she was beginning to connect with her world and the real world. There was promise in the fact that she had learned about the seeds in her class and brought this new knowledge to her therapy session. She had done the same with the chrysalis theme some months before, something we both felt she would have been unable to do a year ago.

The seasons were changing and Amber may have remembered the advent of winter as a time when the weather was getting colder and she did not have the protection of warm clothes. She had also been attending the unit for a year; perhaps she was wondering how long she would remain before a change occurred. The reappearance of the theme of mucous had been interesting. This time she seemed able to externalize her feelings and from this she had moved into a role play which allowed me to understand the abuse that had happened.

The sycamore seeds were sorted into categories and she had asked whether she was good. Most children have a clear understanding of the concept of good and bad and we both felt that Amber was struggling to fit the effects of abuse, both emotional and sexual, within this framework. The play with the seeds where the inside of a seed became 'snot' seemed to illustrate the point.

The role play, and the fact that age was mentioned, was significant. Amber was dealing with the pain and guilt produced by the abuse. She was trying to rationalize that the abuser was older than she, a child, was and therefore knew better, yet the power he had exerted over her made her doubt that he was in the wrong. She was not sure what sort of life he would have in prison and was convinced he had a key for his cell. I had to provide a commentary for this rather than a reflection because I felt she was still powerless. This element of powerlessness is often seen in abused children as they struggle to understand how they have been so horribly hurt both physically and mentally. The abuser may try to coerce the child into thinking that she is at fault, and that being abused is normal. The child's pain and her subsequent feelings do not match the abuser's act or words, and so the child is in turmoil.

The role play was spontaneous and this is often seen in play therapy. It was not directed by the therapist, although I had to think what it meant to Amber and try to help her to externalize what she was feeling to allow an emotional healing to take place. By using dolls as the children and herself and the therapist as the adults, Amber had questioned what had occurred in her past. We knew that Alan had abused her, telling her that he was ill and that the abuse was a way to get him better. We knew that Dr Anderson was the forensic paediatrician who had examined Amber. We both felt that as Amber was beginning to deal with the emotional trauma of the abuse she was able to think more about what had happened. She was sorting out the events in her mind in the same way as she and I had been sorting out the sycamore seeds. The difficulty was that, in order to sort out good from bad, you needed to know how to tell the difference. This could be done with the seeds by seeing how they flew. It is impossible to tell a bad adult from a good one, particularly when the good one is a loved figure. The fact that most child sexual abuse offences are perpetrated by adults who know the child makes it harder for the child to sort out her feelings.

The gender of the therapist

The therapist and child should, if possible, be well matched and this raises the question of the gender of the therapist. Many people who have been abused by a man will ask for a female therapist because they find it easier to relate to someone of a different sex from that of the perpetrator, or because they think someone of the same sex as themselves, as the victim, will understand their feelings better. However, the relationship which develops within the therapy is the key factor and, generally, the genders of the child and the therapist are secondary to the process. It is also important that the child experiences a positive relationship with someone of the same gender as the perpetrator of the abuse. Children in this situation need to learn that not all men are abusers and that not all mothers are cruel; by forming relationships based on trust Amber was learning what relationships could be like, in contrast to the relationships she had known so far. She had told me that her mother had thrown tapes at her and she had begun to compare that with the relationship she had with me, as the therapist; I was a different person although I was an adult, too. Amber verbalized some strong feelings towards me and they were accepted; she was given unconditional positive regard and she began to understand this. Her internal model for relationships underwent a transformation as she formed relationships that had some of the same components as those from her past.

During the next session there were mixed references to the invasion of horrible things into and onto the body, and to elements of parenting. Amber covered her arms in wet sand and she called it 'yukky.' There was magic in the family and this helped to mend things. The session ended with the feeding bottle. The child psychiatrist asked if I felt I had apologized rather than reflected Amber's feelings about finishing the session when she had been lying feeding from the bottle. This may have been the reason she suddenly talked about magic and 'flew' out of the room. I agreed and we both acknowledged that supervision was useful in helping to highlight any issues arising from a session that had been missed or overlooked.

We understood Amber's difficulty in seeing babyhood as a good experience, although she was trying through role play to have a sense of some of it being an enjoyable experience. Magic remained an important influence in being able to make things work or be fixed. This also related to her stage of development where magic does exist, for example, children her age often believe in the tooth fairy. Amber had also shown another developmental trait when revisiting areas of life that she had missed out on as a baby and toddler. The child psychiatrist noted that Amber had had the resources to cope with the bereavement and loss of leaving her mother. We also noted that Amber was now far less aggressive and impulsive in the unit. There was a gradual reduction in her bed wetting and she was beginning to apply herself more consistently to her classwork, and to accept praise for tasks she completed.

9 From green to red

MOVING ON

I walked over to the group room to collect Amber for her session. She was waiting for me by the group room door.

'Is it my turn for OT?' Amber asked.

'Yes, it's after juice time and I have come to see you for your OT.'

Amber came out of the room with me and asked, 'Can we play outside?'

'It is fine to play outside but we shall need our coats and gloves to keep us warm.'

'Let's be in the butterfly world, pretend that we are butterfly children and collect all the jewels. We will be butterfly children and collect the crystals.'

Amber grabbed her coat, hastily put it on and moved into the world of the butterfly children. She ran towards the tennis court and began to pick up the half-frozen leaves and sort out the ice crystals that had formed overnight.

'Look, these have pieces of grass in them, this one has some mud, and this one has some seeds.'

'It seems that some of them are different to the others.'

'Let's lay them out. Pretend that we have wings like a butterfly has. We can use our wings to move them along. Let us collect some more.'

'We need to collect more and move some along. I wonder if you are thinking that you will soon be moving along?'

'Get those ones. I'm not worried. I'll miss the staff but they'll miss me too.'

'Yes, Amber, the staff *will* miss you and will think about you once you have left the unit.'

Amber began to pretend to fly about.

'We don't know the names of things, do we Rick? What is this?' she said, holding a leaf. 'What is this for?' to a ball on the ground.

She played the game for 10 minutes, calling to me to guess the name of things or to describe what different things were for. She was smiling during the game.

It was time to go and we 'flew' back to the group room.

'NIEFS' AND 'BICKS'

The next time that I went to collect Amber she was again waiting by the door of the group room.

'Who have you come for?'

'For you, it's your time to come to OT.'

'Can we go outside?'

'Yes, but we need to put our coats and gloves on because it is very cold today.'

We both ran toward the tennis court.

'We are the butterfly children and we don't know anything.'

'You want us to be the butterfly children who don't know anything. What shall we do?'

'We shall pick up things and give them names. Look, what is this?'

She pulled a face and looked quizzically at the leaf.

'I think it's a "nief." Let it be called a nief,' Amber said.

She suddenly stopped rushing around and said to me, 'My grandfather gave me this. It was my grandmother's,' as she showed me a gold ring.

'You're showing me a gold ring that your grandfather gave to you.'

'Yes, he gave it to me. It's precious and from him.'

'It's from someone in your family and it seems important to you.'

'He is my grandfather. That is why he gave it to me.'

'He's a member of your family which is why he gave you something precious.'

'What's this?' Amber cried, pointing to a stick covered in mud. 'Shall we call it a "bick"?'

'I think that it is hard to talk about some things and it is easier to talk about them if you call them something else.'

'I think it is a stick,' she replied.

I again wondered out aloud if the butterfly world was a safe world where things were called different names from the world where things were real.

As the session progressed we pretended to fly about in the cold winter air, choosing various objects to look at and name or rename. At the end of the session we returned to the warmth of the unit.

OUT INTO THE WORLD

The next week when I went to collect Amber from the group room, she was by the door. As she saw me she ran away from the group room along the corridor towards the playroom. I ran after her. Amber stopped by the gymnasium.

'Do you want to go into the gym? We can go in but we might have to leave because it is the older children's class's turn. If Mrs Newton comes along we will have to go into the playroom.'

Once in the gym Amber started to pretend to fly about. 'Let's fly around.' 'I am the person with knowledge. I know what school is for and I know about the world and everything. I will go to a new school soon.'

'Yes, you will be moving from here soon, and it might be a little strange. Here you know everyone and soon you will move to somewhere you do not know. But you will be able to remember here whenever you want to and perhaps you will come back to see people.'

'Yes, I can come and visit. Look, there's something. What is it? I think it is a "brair".'

Amber looked in puzzlement at the chair. We were then interrupted as the adolescent group came to the gym with their teacher. We knew we would have to move and, as we walked out of the gym, Amber asked if we could go outside. Once outside Amber made her way to the bushes and began to climb up into the branches which were about a metre from the ground. As she sat in the branches I was able to stand close by her.

'I will be going soon. Did my father die?'

I replied that she would be leaving soon and she wondered what had happened to her biological father.

'What do you think happened to him, Amber?'

'I think he died of old age'

'Would you like me to find out how he died? Children often feel sad when someone dies. Sometimes they wonder what their life may have been like if their father had looked after them. Do you ever think that?'

'Sometimes. Perhaps you could be my father?'

'You sometimes think that things would have been different if your dad had lived and that may make you feel cross or sad. You think I could be your dad. It is very sad when we meet people and they cannot be what we want them to be. Your real dad is dead and Alan was not nice to you, but lots of people like you and your grandparents love you.'

It was time to go and we walked back into the comfort of the unit. Instead of going to the green group Amber turned the other way and walked towards the red group.

'Green group told me to go to red group because there are a few nurses off sick.'

As we walked into red group the nurses welcomed her and said that she would be with them for the day because the unit was short-staffed due to illness.

THINKING ABOUT FATHER

When I next went to collect Amber I went towards red group as I knew that she had told the nursing staff that she was too big to stay in green group and that she wanted to stay in red group. She wanted the same named nurse and had told her that she would visit her from red group. As I entered red group Amber looked up and smiled. She was dressed in a costume that she had made. It was a butterfly costume with large brightly coloured wings. She came out of the room and asked to go out onto the tennis court. Here she spent the session flying about and asking me to do the same. We talked of the wonderful world that the butterfly children were in and how we were still learning what was what. Her wings blew in the cool air as she 'flew' about the yard. In the middle of this time I said to Amber,

'Do you remember that I said last time that I would find out about your father?'

Amber nodded her head as she flew past me.

'Would you like me to tell you now or shall we go and sit in the playroom?'

Amber flew towards the bushes where she had first asked me about her father.

'Tell me here,' she said.

I walked towards the bushes as she climbed up and said that I had asked the child psychiatrist about her father and she said that he had not died of old age but in a car crash. Amber looked sad and gazed at me intently. 'Sometimes when people die we feel sad or cross or have some other feelings about them. Sometimes it helps to talk to people and to have a photograph of the dead person.'

We talked about her feelings for a while before I asked, 'Do you have a photograph of your father?'

'Yes, it's at my grandad's house.'

'Perhaps you could ask him to send you a copy of it or get one when you go to stay there.'

'I'm going there at half-term, I think.'

'You think you're going there at half-term. Shall I ask your nurse to find out and tell you the days? Perhaps you can make a calendar to help you know when you are going.'

Amber nodded and climbed out of the tree and ran towards the swings.

'Will you push me?'

'Of course I will. Shall I push you from the front or the back?'

'The back and push me high.'

'We have 5 minutes left before it's time to go back. Is that high enough?'

'No, higher!' she cried.

The session ended and we returned to the group room.

THE TOADSTOOL

The next time that I saw Amber we went straight to the playroom. As we walked in Amber told me that she had made a calendar with her named nurse and that she had been to her aunt's friend's house, a lady who had a beautiful cat named Kali. I reflected that she had sorted out the visit to her grandparents and that her aunt's friend had a cat that Amber liked.

'Yes, she sits on my lap and lets me stroke her. It's lovely when she purrs.' Amber was not doing anything at this time except standing talking. Then she asked if we could go to the pottery room. We made our way to the pottery room and Amber took an apron from the door and went over to the clay. She picked out a piece of clay and, pointing to another child's work, asked if she could make a similar toadstool shape.

'Yes, you can make a toadstool shape. Shall I show you how to make it?'

She nodded and we set about making the toadstool shape.

As she rolled out the clay Amber talked of baking bread with her aunt and how rolling the clay out was similar to working with the dough. She asked about drawing the circle shape for the toadstool lid and decided to use the plastic glass shape to trace around.

I commented that she had a lot of ideas today.

'Yes, I know how to do lots of things. Some of them I have just learned to do and some of them I have known how to do for a long time. Can I take this home when I have finished with it? I will not see my mum, but I will give it to my aunt Marg.'

'You seem sad that you can't take this to your mum but you can give it to your aunt Marg instead.'

'Mmm. My mum can't look after me properly.'

'It is very hard when your mum can't look after you properly and you have to live with other people.'

'Can I paint it red when it's finished?'

'Of course you can,' I replied.

As she sat and finished making the toadstool she talked about her visits to Brownies and the Red Cross group that she belonged to. Her conversation was about the day-to-day events in her life at the present time. When it was time to go Amber had finished her model and placed it on the bench to await firing.

CLINICAL SUPERVISION

I met with the child psychiatrist and we discussed the sessions with Amber since we had last met. In the first of these sessions Amber had returned to the butterfly world, with its themes of crystals, jewels and objects having different names from their names in the real world. This return to earlier material had been a puzzle until I made the link that Amber was thinking about the fact that she would be leaving the unit soon. The child psychiatrist wondered if Amber was preparing to miss the therapist and had thought how she would manage in the world where everything was different to what she had known in the unit. It seemed that by not acknowledging the change in our relationship Amber had taken flight into the butterfly world where she 'flew' about, making therapy difficult as there was no dialogue between us.

Amber had been waiting outside a second time, perhaps unsure if the end of her time in the unit had come. The session was spent outside in the butterfly world, the only dialogue being about her grandfather and the ring she had been given, so her thoughts of separation from the unit may have been particularly strong. The child psychiatrist pondered that the link with the real world was a positive one with talk of Amber's family and of objects, like the ring, that had been given to her. By talking about her grandfather and the ring she may have been telling the therapist that she was capable of forming links with others and that there were other precious things outside of therapy.

The butterfly world appeared in the third session as well and this time allowed another thought to be spoken out loud, namely how Amber's father had died. It was also a return to earlier material and served as a way of stepping out of therapy to ask and receive a direct question and answer. The swirling about between the worlds allowed Amber to discuss the real changes that would soon occur in her life and to reflect upon some events from her past. In the butterfly world everything is nice, in sharp contrast to the real world where very painful thoughts are felt. The session and its content also indicated that Amber was still in a very fragile emotional state and needed space. The outside play area allowed physical expression of this need, in the same way that the gymnasium did. Amber was also telling me that she needed a space away from the intensity of the playroom.

The child psychiatrist and I noted the real change in Amber, her ability to talk more about the life she was living and the events that occurred in it. We also noted the fact that she was preparing to move on and the sense that real emotional growth had occurred. When Amber used the shortage of nursing staff to move into the red group for older children, who were the same age as she was, she was giving out a positive message about herself. She had perceived that she had grown up into the 9-year-old she was chronologically.

The time when Amber made the wings was seen by both of us as true growth. She had become the butterfly all of us had hoped was there. However, the butterfly was still fragile and could be damaged easily. The child psychiatrist noted that Amber was very stressed when in the unit and some of the nursing group thought she might be depressed, although there was no formal sign of this.

The moving about outside while in a therapy session could have occurred for many reasons. The child psychiatrist and I talked about the way Amber was able to create objects with the clay and how she was starting to be as creative as any other 9-year-old child. Gone was the need to use the clay to express her primitive feelings and work out the good from the bad. Instead, I was describing a child who was talking about going to Brownies and the Red Cross group while making a gift for her aunt Marg.

In the nursing group, Amber had matured noticeably and was able to help a girl younger than herself, who was new to the unit, to settle in. In class she completed more written work and her wetting had stopped almost completely. Amber had talked about her brother and sister very sadly and prepared for her contact with them with quiet but eager anticipation. She also seemed to look forward to visits to her grandparents but continued to reflect on the loss of her mother.

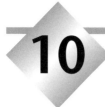

Case review

A case review was held in the child psychiatry department 1 year after the original case discussion. It was attended by the same people as before. It was not expected that Katherine would attend.

UNIT AND COMMUNITY REPORTS

After welcoming everyone to the meeting, the social worker acting as chairman explained that the case had been to court and a 4-day hearing held. Katherine was vigorously represented by a barrister who had fought hard to retain care of all three of the children but this had been rejected by the judge, who had also decided that gradually reducing the level of meetings, with the aim of ending contact with her mother altogether, was in Amber's best interests. Amber had been having regular contact with her paternal grandfather and his second wife and seemed to have had positive experiences on these occasions. They had now applied for Amber to be placed in their care and they had been assessed for this.

The chairman asked for reports from the unit first and then for reports from the community. At present Amber remained with her foster parents. She had had no contact with her mother for the last 3 months but continued to see her siblings on a fortnightly basis. She had also been having regular visits to her grandparents.

The foster mother

An account of Amber's behaviour in foster care was given by her foster mother, who said that there had been a considerable change in Amber who at times could be quite difficult and assertive. She gave an example of how she had made arrangements to take Amber out for a picnic, an activity which Amber normally enjoyed, but when asked to get a jacket in case it rained, she had refused and insisted on wearing a thick jumper only and after a brief argument had sat on the stairs and said she would rather not go than have to wear a jacket. The foster mother said that a compromise had been reached and they had all enjoyed the day out, but she now regarded Amber as behaving more like other girls of her age. The foster mother said that Amber still seemed to be in another world at times but this was far less frequent than previously and, if asked, she would now say that she was thinking about her mother or about when she was younger. She never went into details but would tolerate her foster mother sitting quietly with her at some of these times, although it was clear that really she preferred to be alone.

Amber had continued to eat well and now slept soundly most nights, although she still wet her bed about once per month, often following a period of being preoccupied and sad. The foster mother said that she had not been aware of Amber masturbating in the last month and she had not behaved inappropriately while in her care. She added that Amber now played outside with the other children in the neighbourhood several times a week. This was never for more than an hour at the most and she remained on the periphery of the group, but she had been very pleased when a child had called for her the previous week. Amber's foster father said that he had been very pleased when Amber asked him to teach her to ride a bike, and he had been surprised how quickly she had learned. He said that he and Amber shared an interest in gardening and now she often helped him in the garden.

The social worker

The social worker reported that she took Amber to see Craig and Jenny every 2 weeks. She said that Amber seemed eager to see them and this was confirmed by the foster mother. The social worker said that the children spent 2 hours together in the home of Jenny and Craig's foster mother and seemed to enjoy each other's company. She said that she had noticed that during the last three visits Amber had seemed less anxious about asking them if they were all right, although she remained very affectionate and rather parental in her play with them, taking responsibility for organizing games and mediating disputes. The social worker added that Katherine was sent photographs of the children at regular intervals. All three of the children were aware of this and Amber had checked that her mother had received the photographs at the last contact visit.

The named nurse

Amber's special nurse in the child psychiatry unit reported that Amber continued to have a close relationship with her, but that she had become more involved in friendships with other children in her group and was now content to spend significant periods of time with them without her nurse. Amber had found it difficult when children in her group were discharged from the unit and she had seen this happen a number of times as she had been attending for a long time. When someone left, Amber always made a card for the child and asked very carefully where the child was going and what would be happening to him or her. Amber had become very angry when a new child in the group had asked her if she had a mother and had responded that of course she did, 'the best in the world'.

The unit teacher

Amber's teacher said that Amber was now attending class on a regular basis with two other members of her group. She said that Amber was a very mature member of the group and had become very good at making remarks that stopped others being silly when she wanted to learn something. There were still days when Amber found it very hard to sit still and concentrate, and on these days the teacher had found it better to do practical activities, such as growing plants which remained a favourite for Amber. Amber still produced very little written work but with the aid of the computer had written a number of short essays. The themes of these had concerned children vanquishing evil forces and then dying or being abandoned. Amber loved to be read stories or, failing this, read herself and recently she had started to read to another child younger than herself.

The occupational therapist

Amber's occupational therapist reported that themes from their sessions had included an identification of good and bad, and a need to banish that which was bad. He said that Amber had played out themes which had allowed her to externalize her feelings and she had gone on to banish bad things from the therapy setting. Amber had been more explicit about Alan and prison, and had been able to handle these very emotive issues in a surprisingly resilient way. There had been times when she had returned to themes from the past and reworked the feelings associated with, for example, how her father had died. Amber had also reflected on other members of her family, such as her sister and brother and her grandparents. More recently she had started to think about leaving the child psychiatry unit and her foster parents.

The junior child psychiatrist

The junior child psychiatrist said that he had had a relatively peripheral role in the team but had seen Amber on a regular if infrequent basis. His task had been mostly to monitor her mental state and also to act as case manager, ensuring good liaison with other agencies. The doctor said that Amber had not suffered from any formal psychiatric illness during her admission in that, although there had been times when she had been very unhappy and distressed, her mental state had not reached the level of a formal diagnostic category. He said that he had been impressed by the increasing maturity that Amber had shown and that now she was able to talk with him not only about weekly life events but also to reflect a little on the past, and on how it related to her wishes for the future.

The consultant child psychiatrist

The consultant said that she agreed with the junior child psychiatrist's view and she noted that Amber's ability to learn in class and in her nursing group was vastly different from when she was admitted. She was no longer a girl who seemed 'switched off' but, on the contrary, was now fully involved in what was going on around her, was sensitive to the needs of others, had a keen sense of how to assert herself, and did not appear to be cognitively impaired after all. The child psychiatrist added that it seemed that psychologically Amber had grown enormously and the developmental stage that she had reached was now appropriate for her chronological age. She had moved through the various developmental stages rapidly and, although she still moved back and forth in terms of her developmental functioning, this was perhaps only slightly more than a comparable child of her own age. The child psychiatrist also reflected that Amber was a child who had experienced significant trauma on many levels and she would always retain some mark from this. However, it looked as if she would reach a point where these marks were painful memories which she had come to terms with but that did not impair her functioning. Amber had been in the child psychiatry department for a considerable period of time and there were now signs that she was coming to the end of her period there. Amber herself was starting to reflect on issues of leaving and the view of the team working with her was that planning was needed to enable Amber to leave in the not too distant future.

AMBER'S FUTURE CARE

The chairman said that he was very pleased to hear how well Amber was progressing and there was now a need to reach a conclusion about her future care. He introduced Mrs Brown, an independent social worker from Bournemouth. She had undertaken an assessment of Amber's maternal grandparents with regard to their application to care for Amber in the future. The legal situation was that Amber was on a care order in the care of Mr and Mrs Bradley (whom Amber called Aunt Margaret and Uncle Bob).

Mrs Brown had regular contact with Jenny and Craig who were also on care orders and in foster care together with a different family from Amber. Amber, Jenny and Craig had no contact with their mother but she was sent photographs and cards on a regular basis and the children were aware of this. There was no contact with the children's paternal families as it was not known who they were and Amber's father was dead. Katherine's father and stepmother lived in Bournemouth and had only infrequent contact with her and the children after a major disagreement, following which Katherine had moved north. Amber's grandparents had applied for a residence order to allow them to care for Amber. This had been fiercely opposed by Katherine, who had accused her father of never having been interested in her as a child or in Amber as his grandchild.

Mrs Brown reported how she had undertaken her assessment of the grandparents, meeting with them on several occasions and also visiting their home. She offered her opinion that there were a number of concerns about their ability to care for Amber. Firstly there was the question of their relationship with Katherine, which was acrimonious and which had deteriorated further when the grandparents had made an application for a residence order. There was also the question of the quality of parenting that had been given to Katherine when she was a child which could be thought by some to have affected her ability to care for Amber, Jenny and Craig. Mrs Brown was also concerned that Mr and Mrs Wilson had been married for only 5 years and had not had to care for children together. Mrs Wilson was not a relative of Amber's but seemed to have formed a good relationship with her. She had two grown-up children from a previous relationship and had regular and frequent contact with both them and her grandchildren. Mr Wilson seemed to have formed a very good relationship with Amber and he looked forward to and planned for her visits to Bournemouth. He was also having contact with Jenny and Craig and they had all spent a number of afternoons together in Newcastle. Mrs Brown said that Mr and Mrs Wilson were in their 60s and enjoyed reasonably good health. Mr Wilson had had some surgery to his knee from an old sports injury and Mrs Wilson suffered from high blood pressure, but both were active lively people. Overall, the view of Mrs Brown was that, although she had some reservations about Mr and Mrs Wilson having long-term care of Amber, this seemed to offer a reasonable option for the little girl.

The conference members discussed this suggestion in some detail, many expressing the view that, given the very serious concerns about the care that Amber had received, questions must be asked about Mr Wilson's role in looking after her when she was little. Other issues related to Amber's need for long-term stability and the fact that Mr and Mrs Wilson would not normally expect to care for a small child at this stage in their lives. The continued viability of their marriage, given the added dimension of hostility from Katherine and the fact that Amber was not Mrs Wilson's own grandchild, was raised. It was also pointed out that, although Amber had made great progress, she remained a very fragile and vulnerable child who had great needs yet to be met. She was likely to need a considerably greater level of support for a longer period of time than other children who had not had to deal with her life experiences. If Amber did go to Mr and Mrs Wilson and her mother tried to make contact this could prove very difficult for her, particularly if Mr Wilson was ambivalent in his responses to Katherine who he said he still cared for as his daughter. An additional concern was how Jenny and Craig would react to their sister's placement with their grandparents without them.

Amber's own view of what she wanted for the future was one of the most important considerations. Her nurse said that Amber always looked forward to her grandparent's visits and, whereas at first this related more to her pleasure at seeing Craig and Jenny, she felt that Amber now genuinely wanted to see her granddad and grandma. After she had seen the Wilsons, either with or without her brother and sister, she was often very excitable and wanted to talk about all the exciting things they had done. The nurse pointed out that this was a false situation as everyday life did not consist of a continuous round of activities. Amber's teacher said that Amber had gone to Bournemouth to spend 4 days with her grandparents recently and she had prepared for this visit by finding out where Bournemouth was on the map and tracing the route they would drive to get there. She had also wanted to make a trip to the beach near Newcastle to get some idea of the sea life she might find as she knew that her granddad would take her for walks on the beach.

The child psychiatrist said that she had observed Amber with her grandparents on three occasions and she was struck by how relaxed and happy Amber was with her grandfather and how they clearly shared a number of interests. She had noticed that Mrs Wilson seemed a little left out at times but that Mr Wilson and Amber both actively included her when this happened. Amber had been very excited when visiting her siblings with her grandparents, and Jenny and Craig had been upset when Amber 'showed-off' about her trip to Bournemouth. Mr and Mrs Wilson had assured Jenny and Craig that they could come and visit at some time in the future. The child psychiatrist said that she had talked to Amber alone a number of times to review events while she had been a patient and had gone on to explore her wishes about the future. Amber had been very enthusiastic about going to live with her grandparents but had said that if she really could choose she would want to see her mother and perhaps go and live with her in the future. She was very clear that she wanted to see Jenny and Craig often, and was concerned that if she went to Bournemouth and they stayed in Newcastle this would not be possible. She was also concerned about leaving

Aunt Margaret and Uncle Bob and also her friends in the child psychiatry unit. She asked if she could take photographs so that she would 'always remember.'

The conference also considered that an assessment of Amber's educational needs would need to be formalized. The educational psychologist said that his assessment showed that Amber was of average ability and he would liaise with the education services in Bournemouth about Amber's school planning. The view of the team from the child psychiatry unit was that probably she would cope in a mainstream provision but that she was likely to need additional support. This support would be required to help her to integrate into a peer group at a time when she still had to work through a considerable number of psychological issues.

The conference finally agreed to recommend to the court that Amber would be introduced gradually into living at her grandfather's home with a view to making this her home, too. She would maintain regular contact with her siblings, and Mr and Mrs Wilson would be encouraged both to invite Jenny and Craig to visit and to come to Newcastle themselves on a regular basis. Monitoring of the progress of this plan would be undertaken and Mr and Mrs Wilson would be offered support from the social work team to help them to deal with the changes that would follow with Amber moving into their home, and also to help them to support Amber and manage any emotional or behavioural difficulties. Amber would be referred to the local child and adolescent psychiatry department to provide her with psychological support. A statement of special educational needs would be requested.

The local authority solicitor said this would mean that the local authority would be supporting Mr and Mrs Wilson in their application for residence order but would wish to retain a monitoring and supportive role in this case. It was agreed that this was the decision of the case conference and that reports would be prepared by the child psychiatry team, social workers and educational psychologist for use in the court hearing which would be in the next few weeks. The members of the child psychiatry team agreed that Amber would continue to attend the department until she was well integrated into a plan for a move to her grandparents and then would keep in touch with her when she returned to Newcastle on visits.

Placement

The case review meeting was convened as arranged at the previous case conference and all the areas of functioning in Amber's life were reviewed as a routine. One of the guiding principles of the Children Act 1989 (England and Wales) is that wherever possible a child should remain in his or her family of origin but, in this situation, it was not possible for Amber to be cared for safely by her mother and she was placed with a foster family. When her grandparents made it clear that they wanted to care for her the lead agencies considered them very carefully as potential carers, in order to avoid Amber being removed totally from her family.

The various concerns about this placement are of the type that often arise in a situation where a child remains in the care of the extended family. It can be a very complex situation, requiring a great deal of care, support and careful monitoring, to ensure that the child's needs are being met. Not only did decisions need to be made about where Amber would live but also whether or not a legal order was required. In addition, decisions regarding contact with her mother and other members of the family had to be made, and these would need to be held under review.

11

Goodbye

A DOG FOR AUNT MARG

Amber was half-way down the corridor when I went to collect her.

'It's my turn for OT. Come on, hurry up,' she said, enthusiastically.

She ran towards the activities unit and stopped outside the pottery room door.

'Would you like to go and see if your toadstool is ready for glazing or painting?' I asked.

She nodded and opened the door. Amber quickly saw that the pottery model had been fired and was waiting to be glazed.

'Can it be red?' she asked. I reminded her that it could be any colour and that we had said it could be red last time.

I opened the door to the cupboard and showed Amber the paint and glazes that were there, explaining as I did so that each object required three coats of the colour to work properly. Amber picked up one of the pots and read out the colour.

'"Moroccan Brown," "Canary Yellow," "Novelty Red." Is this the one Rick?'

I said that it was and that it was called 'Novelty Red' because it was only for ornaments and the glaze could not be used for cups or plates that may contain liquid or food. We selected the paint brushes and Amber began to paint.

'Why is it pink?'

I explained that the glaze became red in the kiln but as a liquid it was pink.

'Does it get very hot in the kiln?'

'Yes it goes up to 1000 degrees Celsius.'

Amber asked if that was very hot and I said that it was.

'How long will it take before I can collect it? Can I have it this afternoon?'

I said I knew she was keen to collect the toadstool as soon as possible and perhaps she was worried that it may be left behind when she left the unit. I also said that because the kiln was so hot it would not be ready until tomorrow.

'Do things get left behind?' asked Amber, as she looked up to the shelf which contained a number of fired and glazed objects.

'No, children decide what they want to do with their things. Some children want to leave the things they have made, some want to give them to people, others do different things with their models. When you leave you can decide what you want to do with anything that you have made.'

'Will I come back?'

'Yes, you will come back to visit and say hello, but you do not need to come every week as some children you have known do. Things are very different from when you first came and soon you will be leaving to live with your grandparents.'

'They speak funny,' said Amber.

As she carefully painted the toadstool with the three coats, we spoke about accents and the slight uncertainty that moving to a new house would bring. Amber asked me about taking the toadstool home and I reassured her that there was plenty of time and that she knew when she was leaving. I reminded her that there would be a party for her which would be her leaving party.

'Can you come to it?'

'Yes, of course. Sometimes when we leave somewhere we are sad or have other feelings,' I said.

'Have you ever left anywhere?' asked Amber.

'Yes, and sometimes I was sad to leave, but I knew I could visit, write letters or telephone if I wanted.'

'I think that I will visit. What can I do after this?'

We discussed the various options and Amber thought that she could make a plaster of Paris dog.

'Aunt Marg can have this because it will be ready for today.'

I thought aloud that it was important to have something for Aunt Marg.

'Yes, she has a cold today and I want to give her something to make her feel better.'

The plaster of Paris dog took a few minutes to make and as it was drying we cleared up the room.

I mentioned the time and Amber asked to make a box for the dog, which we started to do.

'Aunt Marg will like this, blue is her favourite colour.'

I replied that Amber was keen to give something to Aunt Marg and that the Aunt had a cold. I wondered if Amber was worried about her.

'Will she die?'

'No, not from a cold. Everyone dies some day but not from colds. You will not be left alone. Your Aunt Marg will still be there when you go home. We can telephone her if you wish or I can ask the nurses to let you call her.'

As Amber pulled the mould off and placed the model in the box she asked if she could call her Aunt when she went back to the group room. I said that I would tell the nurses what we had said and someone would go with her. As our time had finished we left the room, with Amber holding the box very tightly.

KEEPING SAFE

When I next went to collect Amber one of the staff told me that she had been told the day that she would leave the unit by the child psychiatrist. All the team had known the day but Amber was not told until it was finalised. Amber was just coming out of class as I arrived at the door. She asked if it was her turn and accompanied me to the activities unit. She said that she wanted to bake, to which I had replied that as long as the kitchen was free she could. Amber looked into the kitchen.

'It's free. Can I get the doll from the playroom?'

Amber rushed off and returned with a doll from the playroom. Amber then said that she was the mother of the doll, which was a little baby. I was to be the social worker and Amber told me to sit down in my office. She placed the doll on the bench and went to get some paper towels to place over the doll informing me that the baby was going to go to sleep. As the baby slept Amber walked around imitating adult life, pretending to clean and wash up.

'What shall I do?' I asked.

'Ssh, you'll wake the baby. You stay in your office until I call you.'

The baby woke up and Amber went over and tried to feed it.

'Ssh little baby, what do you want? Something to eat? Here you are, hungry are you?'

She then said, 'I'll ring you up because a bad man is coming and we have to leave the house. You can help find another house for us.'

The 'telephone' rang and I answered it, 'Hello, social work here. Can I help?'

'Yes, it's Mrs Jewel. Can you get me a new house? Alan is coming out and I need to leave. He might harm the baby.'

'I see. You want a new house because Alan is getting out of prison and you think he may harm the baby. The police have been told to lock him up if he comes near the baby. Shall I come over?'

Amber thought for a few seconds and said, 'Yes, please.'

I stopped the role play and asked Amber if she was worried about something as I knew that Alan had been put in prison. Amber did not reply so I told her that the judge and social services had told Alan that he was not allowed to go near her and if she ever saw him she was to tell whoever she was with that he had been told not to go near her. I acknowledged that Amber may be scared that Alan would come and get her but the police and others knew that he was not allowed to do this. I repeated that what he had done had been wrong.

'I should have told on him,' said Amber.

'You could not have told on him because you were too little and he tricked you. How old were you?'

'About 6.'

'Yes and when you were 6 you were a little girl and he was a grown-up.'

'He was old and should have known better, shouldn't he Rick?'

'Yes, he was wrong to do what he did, but you were little and it is not your fault that you did not tell until later. If ever you do not like something someone else does you should tell an adult. If they don't listen tell another, like a teacher. You will always be believed.'

Amber said nothing but appeared to listen. She picked up the doll and rocked it to and fro.

'It is very difficult to leave a place you like and move to a new place. You have visited your grandparents' house and stayed there and will leave the unit next week to go and live there. They will keep you safe.'

'I will leave on Friday. Dr Kaplan told me today.'

'Yes, you will leave then.'

'Have I got time to make some crispies?'

'Yes. Shall we get the things we need out?'

We spent the rest of the session making some crispies, Amber talking about her Aunt Marg and telling me that she was much better. Just before the end we spoke about having to leave her Aunt's house and how sad she was to do this.

As we packed up the finished crispies in the bag Amber said, 'I think I'll miss OT.'

I replied, 'And OT will miss you.'

STORIES AND SEEDS

As I went to collect Amber from her group room in her last week, I stopped at the door and saw that she was not inside. One of the staff told me that she was in class and would be out in a minute. Amber appeared seconds later.

'I told Miss that it was my OT time and I was waiting for you to come and collect me.'

I laughed and said, 'And I'm waiting to collect you. We are both waiting.'

Amber went into the pottery room and picked up her glazed toadstool (Fig. 11.1). She thought that it looked beautiful and held it close to her body.

'Aunt Marg will love this.'

She moved out of the room into the playroom and having carefully placed the object on the table sat on the beanbag.

'Can I have a story and some juice?'

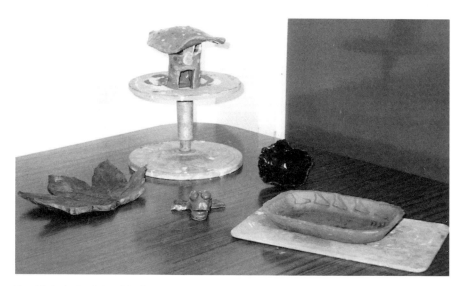

Fig. 11.1 Amber's toadstool.

As I nodded, Amber went to fill the feeding bottle and asked for *Cinderella* to be read to her. She settled herself on the beanbag and drank from the bottle as I read the story. As the story finished I mentioned that we would have this time and next time together and after that Amber would leave the unit.

'Can I have another story? The Gingerbread Man.'

As I read the story, Amber joined in with the chorus of 'Run, run, as quick as you can. You can't catch me, I'm the gingerbread man.'

Amber lay on the beanbag and finished her drink. She wanted *Cinderella* to be reread and then changed her mind.

'Can we get the sycamore seeds out?'

I lifted the box down and Amber started to categorize the various seeds and throw them in the air. As they fell she sorted them out.

'That's a bad one,' and she quickly split it open revealing the green seed. 'Put it in the bin, it's a bad one.'

She threw a number of seeds into the air and all the bad ones were placed in the bin.

'Let's hit them really hard,' she said, as she hit the top of the container with a wooden spoon.

'Ha, ha! They're all going away. What a headache they will have. Look, Rick! The bad ones are all going away. They will never come back, never.'

'You're hitting all the bad ones and they will never come back. You're hitting them so hard that they will never, ever come back.'

'Yes, throw them all away.'

She then threw the container into the rubbish bin.

'Can I wrap up Aunt Marg's gift?'

As we had a few minutes we found some tissue paper and wrapped up the gift. Just before we finished I repeated that the next session would be the last one.

'You've told me that already, silly,' replied Amber, as she walked out the door. We walked over to the group room door and one of the nurses said that the others were having an early lunch because there was an outing that afternoon to the beach. Amber smiled at the thought of playing on the sand and ran off towards the canteen.

THE LAST OT SESSION

When I next walked towards the group room door another child from Amber's group asked if I would sign the leaving card that the group had made for her, which I did. Amber was waiting by the door when I appeared.

'Whose turn is it for OT?'

'It is your turn. Would you like to come along?'

As we walked towards the playroom, Amber said that this was going to be the last time that she would walk towards OT. I agreed and as we went into the playroom said that she sounded a little sad.

'Yes, it is so sad when everything has to end. OT is my own time and now it's going.'

I reflected that the time had been important and that she would have memories of me and others on the unit. I wondered if she would like to use the Polaroid camera to take some pictures of the room and of me. I suggested that she would be able to place them in the life-story book that she and her social worker had been working on.

'Can I? Where is the camera?'

As I showed her the camera and how it worked she got ready to take my picture.

'Stand there, Rick.'

The photographic images came out and Amber was amazed. Soon she had a small pile of pictures of the room she had used. I asked if she would like to say goodbye to any of the other rooms that she had used.

'No, thanks,' she replied. 'I just want to sit here and blow some bubbles.'

She sat on the small chair and I passed her the bubble blower. Amber sat and blew large multicoloured bubbles into the room. She tried to blow the biggest, the smallest and the most at once.

'I'm going to live with my grandparents. They live a long way away.'

I repeated back to Amber that things were changing, that she was soon to go and live with her grandparents and that they did live a long way away. We thought together how she might remember Aunt Marg and other people she had met in the past 2 years. Some of the ideas were to telephone and to write letters.

Amber said that she wanted to write down the address and telephone numbers of the unit. I found her a piece of paper and together we made a little booklet in which she wrote the names of people she knew and the telephone number. I reminded her that her grandparents and social worker would have the number if she lost her booklet. It was time to go and we walked towards the group room.

'Goodbye, Rick. Will you be at my party?'

'Goodbye, Amber. Yes, of course I will be at your party.'

LEAVING PARTY

The next day was Amber's last day and the group had been busy making cakes and decorating the room. Cards were signed and bunting hung up. Amber was being collected by her grandparents and Aunt Marg after lunch. Amber spent the morning in class and had a little time to say goodbye to her named nurse and other people and children whom she knew.

The time for Amber's leaving party came and all the group participated in the ritual. Some presents were given and party games played. Amber sat in the middle of it all, sometimes participating and sometimes looking thoughtful, perhaps thinking of the future where her peers would be a normal school population, something she had often longed for. I spent a little time in the room but having said my goodbyes left quietly as the party ended and class, OT and group resumed for the last 1¼ hours of the timetable prior to lunch.

Giving gifts

There are differing views about the giving of cards and presents by the therapist. Some people feel it is a normal activity and part of the way we say goodbye to people. Others feel that the relationship which has been built up between child and therapist is what counts and is what the child will carry away with her. Many therapists do not give gifts because the gifts may break or be destroyed and this may leave the child with feelings of a broken, incomplete relationship. I do not give presents although the taking of photographs can be seen as a kind of gift. It remains a personal decision for each therapist. The important thing to remember is to do what the child wants not what you want. Some therapists feel it is difficult to say goodbye and shower the child with gifts. I wonder what message this gives to the other children who may not get the same gift?

CLINICAL SUPERVISION

Later that day I met with the child psychiatrist and we discussed the last sessions of therapy. Amber had been able to verbalize the ending of her time at the unit and reflect upon it. She had wondered about returning to the unit and had made plans to keep in contact. The photos would go into her life-story book which was a record of her life so far. She would be able to look at the book as often as she wanted to. However, she had been concerned about her foster mother to the point of worrying if she would die, so she still became anxious very easily.

The play about finding a new home for the baby reflected her own move but also made some old worries reappear: was Alan going to be released from prison and then come to track her down? She had doubts that the abuse was all his fault and wavered in her own mind as to whose fault it was. There was some returning to old material, the sycamore seeds, but this time there was a sense of getting rid of the bad ones.

Many people had worked with Amber and her siblings, and a period of intense work was nearing completion. The next phase would be overseen by the social services adoption and fostering unit. Our feeling was that Amber needed to be seen briefly in a child and family psychiatry setting for a limited period of time, perhaps during the settling-in period, and that further intervention might be needed when she became an adolescent. Her grandparents were aware of this and had spoken to the child psychiatrist about their worries for Amber's future, especially her ability to build a loving and eventually sexual relationship with a person of her choice when she became old enough.

The child psychiatrist and I spoke about our own feelings of loss that were surfacing in knowing that Amber was leaving. It was hard for everyone to say goodbye and the staff hoped that Amber would take with her an invisible suitcase full of the good experiences she had had, into which she could dip when life became difficult. Such a suitcase is our hope for the future of every child with whom we work. We were aware that this optimism was fragile, and that there were doubts that Amber would be able to go to mainstream school or be able to adjust to living without the support of the various people and agencies who had been part of her life over the past few years.

Now that her therapy was over, we decided to reflect upon the management of Amber and this is dealt with in the next chapter.

12 Conclusion

PSYCHODYNAMIC THEORY (AINSCOUGH & TELFORD 1995)

Although Axline's framework for non-directive therapy guides therapists in what they should say and do (Axline 1989), it does not explain
what happens within therapy sessions as regards the interaction and
responses of the child. It is more a formula for use than a philosophy
underpinning the therapeutic process, and it focuses on the therapist
rather than the child. In order to develop a more comprehensive understanding of the child, clinicians tend to adopt a second but compatible
theoretical framework, that of psychodynamic theory.

A trusting relationship

In order to understand fully the therapeutic process we decided to match
the time Amber spent in therapy with the existing theories (Table 12.1).
The most important aspect of therapy is to develop a warm and friendly
relationship with the child; this is central to both non-directive and
psychoanalytical therapy. The relationship can be understood as being
similar to the first one the child had, namely with her mother. Apart
from physical needs, a baby requires emotional warmth, synchronicity
and containment to establish a sense of safety and trust in a relationship.
Motivated by a sense of empathy and a desire to alleviate distress, the
parent tunes in to the signals given by the baby and, having an idea of
the cause of stress, can do something to change the situation, i.e. provide a feed or change the nappy. The baby gains something more than
physical satisfaction from this action. Having experienced pain or a
sense of discomfort, for which the cause or origin is as yet incomprehen-
sible, the baby cries; the parent's response in alleviating the pain and

Table 12.1 Theories of personality development				
	Freud	**Erikson**	**Piaget**	**Social play**
1st year	Oral stage	Trust versus mistrust		Solitary mother/child
2nd year	Anal stage	Autonomy versus shame and doubt	Sensorimotor (0–2 years)	Mother/child parallel
3rd to 5th years	Phallic stage	Initiative versus guilt	Preoperational (2–7 years)	Looking on and cooperative
6th year to puberty	Latency period	Industry versus inferiority	Concrete operational (7–12 years)	Cooperative and formal
Adolescence	Genital stage	Identity versus confusion	Formal operational (over 12 years)	
Early adulthood		Intimacy versus isolation		
Middle adulthood		Generativity versus self-absorption		
Ageing years		Integrity versus despair		

attendant distress communicate to the baby both that her environment is, on the whole, congenial and not life threatening, and that she can weather the machinations of pain, albeit only for a short time at first.

The therapeutic situation attempts to recreate this pattern of communication in order to develop a trusting and child-centred relationship. The therapist offers a professional understanding of child development through theoretical training and a knowledge of the intrapsychic world of the child (that is, the internal workings of the child's mind). The situation is more complex when dealing with children rather than babies however, because there are other factors involved which make the establishment of a trusting relationship alone insufficient to meet their needs.

Communicating through play

The channels of communication available to a child are more varied and sophisticated than those of a baby. Children have experienced formative and deformative life events, and learned coping strategies which affect their thoughts, feelings and behaviour. Alongside a trusting relationship the therapist needs to develop a good rapport with the child. A child's natural form of communication is through play. Winnicott believed that to 'stop playing is to stop thinking' (Winnicott 1971). Play is the vehicle by which rapport is established. Given a trusting relationship in an environment which facilitates communication, the therapist invests in the child's ability to play to express her inner world. In relation to Amber, the vehicle of play allowed some insight into her inner world and there were numerous examples of her having developed a friendly relationship with the therapist. In order to help Amber further, the therapist had to be alert to 'recognize the feelings the child is expressing and reflecting them back in such a manner that some insight into their behaviour was gained' (Axline 1989).

The therapist had to learn to identify emotions from Amber's non-verbal communication, and then reflect them back to her as a range of possibilities as to how she might be feeling. This represented an attempt to open communication and reach an understanding of Amber. Amber used this link to begin to make sense of her internal and external world. Gaining this insight required effort on the part of Amber and the therapist because all the different elements of thought, feeling, behaviour and life events which have to be linked together are not necessarily readily available in the conscious of the child.

The conscious consists of the thoughts and feelings of which the child is currently aware. The other end of this continuum is the unconscious, the domain of life 'instincts' which embody basic life energies like hunger. The mediator between the conscious and the unconscious is the preconscious, the area in which acceptable thoughts and feelings are stored because it would be impossible for every thought and feeling to impinge on the conscious at the same time. When defence mechanisms as described by Freud (1915) operate they protect the child from intrapsychic conflict and, thus, their influence extends across the conscious, preconscious and unconscious as channels for thoughts and feelings. Defence mechanisms help reduce anxiety and are usually unconscious, for example repression, but if the therapist accurately reflects the affect of the child it is likely that he is tapping into information stored in the preconscious. By making these feelings conscious, the child has the opportunity to explore the link between that particular feeling and the behaviour which provoked it. The process of matching thought, behaviour and emotion results in insight and understanding.

The therapist must allow a degree of permissiveness so the child can express her real feelings. In setting limits of behaviour while being non-judgmental, the therapist encourages an atmosphere of freedom, of being able to express anything, however difficult or upsetting. For the child, the room and the therapist become associated in a dynamic link known as containment.

The idea of containment is underpinned by the concept of holding. The therapist 'holds' the session together both on a practical level and in his own mind. He acts as an emotional container because he experiences and keeps within himself the emotions of the child without being overwhelmed by them; he can therefore take control of them in a non-defensive way. The powerful feelings felt by the therapist during Amber's play in the 'snots and smearing' play illustrate this (p. 51).

The analytical concept of transference, as the traditional psychodynamic method of externalizing and resolving intrapsychic conflict, was also at work in Amber's relationship with the therapist. Transference occurs when the infant prototypes reemerge and are experienced with a strong sense of immediacy; in other words, the child replicates the dynamics of a past relationship in the present with the therapist. The process of transference almost always operates in a therapeutic relationship and it is the dynamics of past relationships which remain unresolved and troublesome that will be communicated in this way. If these feelings are contained and then acknowledged, they become externalized and available to the conscious of the child. It is then possible for a resolution of these feelings to occur, as was seen when Amber was cross with the therapist for going on holiday (p. 88).

The creation of a personality

Another theory we considered to explain the way Amber had presented was that developed by Erik Erikson (1965) in which life was seen as a series of psychosocial developments. Erikson's theory traces the individual creation of self through relationships with others, firstly by introjection and then by identification. Introjection occurs when the child is a baby and involves incorporating another's image, i.e. a parent's image; identification occurs when the child enjoys being like other people, particularly at adolescence. Amber would have introjected the chaos of her mother's personality and based her identity on the significant adults who were around as she grew and developed. Erikson also postulated that we develop through a series of psychosocial stages which ultimately shape our personality.

The lack of trust Amber had displayed and her inability to be autonomous in the routines of her daily life mirrored Erikson's theory. She also lacked a sense of industry and initiative. Through milieu therapy, she moved back into a normal pattern of living, as was seen in the creativity and decision-making she showed in the latter stages of therapy.

Developmental process

A clear developmental process in both motor and cognitive abilities is often seen in play therapy and this was the case with Amber. Children often arrive at therapy some way behind in the developmental process, e.g. their play is that of a younger child, they cannot play cooperatively with other children, or their motor skills are those seen in younger children. Amber could not play cooperatively with the children in her group and her play was that of a younger child when she first arrived on the unit. The structure of the unit, both internally and externally, allows a child the chance to undertake the developmental process at her own pace. The adventure playground, tennis court and grassed area allow freedom of movement, and the milieu of the unit allows freedom of thought.

THE MULTIDISCIPLINARY TEAM

Amber was aided in her recovery by a multidisciplinary team, in which individual professionals contributed a wide variety of skills. The staff at the unit are experts in the mental health of children and young people, and have built up a knowledge-base over some 25 years. The individuals work as a team, trusting and respecting each other. Many share post-professional training in therapies such as systemic family therapy (which sees the family as a system), thus increasing the treatment options available to the children and their families.

The team have a strong belief in the value of supervision and adhere strictly to clear managerial lines. The staff who worked most closely with Amber received their supervision in a variety of ways, including the formal individual sessions described in 'Clinical supervision' and in ward rounds, held on a weekly basis. The ward round allows the management and therapy of each child to be discussed in a multidisciplinary meeting so the staff can reflect upon the feedback from their colleagues. Members of the team are encouraged to attend conferences and training courses to ensure that the children receive the most up-to-date care available. It is important that the team has a strong team leader, in Amber's case the child psychiatrist, who discussed her in the review meetings and who ensured maximum use of the supervision setting. It is also important that all staff are supported by each other to achieve the best therapeutic milieu. For example, if a child has been extremely angry with a member of staff there will always be at least one person to sit with him or her to reflect upon the incident and provide support, if appropriate.

The layout of the unit helps the milieu: outside, Amber had a sense of freedom yet she was surrounded by either a wall or a fence; inside she also had a feeling of freedom and security. Every child is observed at all times by someone, which lessens conflict because staff can intervene quickly. In the case of disputes a witness is always available, creating a sense of security. Communication is very good and all staff regard the children as their prime focus of attention. The management of difficult and disturbed children has to be skilfully carried out and is based on the creation of an atmosphere which helps the children to achieve their potential.

AT HOME AND AT SCHOOL

Any form of work with a child with mental health problems must take into consideration the context in which the child lives. The most important factor to consider is the child's family, as they are the people closest to the child and most involved in her daily care over the period of her childhood. Of course, there are some children who will not be living with their biological families and this means that the multidisciplinary team must consider in what way they can provide help to the birth parents who may have contact with the child, as well as the family with whom the child is currently living. Some children, sadly, will have moved through a number of different care situations, including a number of different foster carers as well as children's homes run by the social services department. This lack of stability makes providing therapy particularly complex and careful planning is needed, as well as clarity about the role of everyone connected with the child.

The parents of a child receiving therapy can have difficulty in handling their own feelings about the situation. They may resent the idea that people are critical of the care they have given to the child and be distressed at the possibility that others can do it better than they can. This form of hostility often remains unspoken but needs to be taken into consideration by any professional working with a child. The parents may also feel that their privacy is being invaded by the probing questions that may be asked, and feel, as Katherine did, a sense of unwarranted interference. Working with parents in the context of child protection is a complex job and it requires sensitivity towards the individuals involved, careful planning, excellent communication and good supervision.

Parents who foster a child receiving therapy can find the situation harder to handle than they might have expected. These parents are usually very experienced, competent parents. However, professionals in the team, backed by their training and knowledge, sometimes feel that the foster parents assume greater competence in understanding complex issues than they should. In addition, foster parents form a relationship with the child in their care and, very naturally, develop strong feelings about the child's past experiences which can affect their attitude to the child's biological parents. Also, many foster parents have a child in their care only for a short term. This can be as difficult for the adults as it is for the child and can result in foster parents having strong views about the next placement for the child. Their views need to be considered but should be evaluated as a part of a wider view involving all the people concerned, not least the child herself.

How the child functions within a neighbourhood is also an important factor in her therapy. In this case, Amber initially made little contact with other children in her street and only later was able to form some friendships. However, if a child is not so reserved and poses a significant source of concern and anger in the community, the situation can be awkward. For example, many children who have been abused, are in care, distressed or upset, may behave in an aggressive and destructive way. They may also behave in a sexualized way, which means that they have to be constantly supervised in peer play in a way that other children may dislike. In addition, parents of other children may be reluctant to let their own children play with a child who has had probems and who, as a result, may raise issues or show behaviour to which they would rather not expose their own children. If a child's history becomes known in a neighbourhood and her behaviour marks her out as different, the other children may tease or bully her and even make life difficult for the children of the family who have offered the child foster care. The child can become very distressed under these circumstances and can exaggerate the sort of behaviour for which she is being victimized.

Similar problems arise at school. Children like Amber often find it difficult to focus on classroom activities and this can lead to the view that they are not very bright, as in Amber's case, when, in fact, they are quite able. The child with problems is so overwhelmed by her life experiences that what goes on in a classroom is almost incidental for her. In addition, difficulties in concentrating as well as some non-compliant behaviour may result in her being chastized by teaching staff, further damaging her fragile sense of self-esteem and giving her classmates ammunition for teasing. Sensitive classroom management, where a child is supported and helped to achieve small successes, can make an enormous difference to a child like Amber. In the playground, the same kind of difficulties as in the home street can arise so close supervision and support is needed.

Schools can be placed under enormous pressure not to provide education for a child who poses significant management problems, particularly where there is a possibility that other children may be exposed to inappropriate sexualized behaviour or aggression from a particular child. Additional support is needed in the classroom and also the playground, and this is expensive and often cannot be made available easily.

The need to formalize a statement of the child's educational needs can be complicated because final decisions about where the child will live can take some time to be made and only a person with parental responsibility can make definitive decisions about the educational provision accepted for a child. Amber is a good example of a child whose educational needs changed over time and, therefore, the provision that would have been made for her when she was first referred was not of the kind that she needed when discharged.

CONCLUSION

Amber was initially put on an interim care order. This allowed the local authority to exercise parental responsibility, as well as allowing Katherine to retain her parental responsibility. At the final hearing, the judge gave a full care order to the local authority thus lifting the time restriction for the exercise of parental authority that applies when the order is an interim one. Following this, consideration of Amber's placement with her grandparents was made and she was ultimately placed with them on a residence order.

The role of the mental health team in child protection can be difficult to define precisely. The skills of the many disciplines involved, at the most specialized level of the health service system, can provide expertise in many areas and in many ways. To concentrate only on those children who have a classifiable form of mental illness is, in our view, to diminish and constrain the benefit to children that can be offered by the team. Our work is primarily related to those who have mental illness but it is far broader in scope, and should relate to identifying those children whose growth and development is being impaired by their life experiences.

The range of interventions which can be offered by the mental health team include psychodynamically oriented therapies, family therapy, behaviour therapy, cognitive therapy, drug therapy and in- and day-patient admissions. The work can take different forms, such as consultation, liaison, and direct work with the child and family. It is important for the mental health team to focus on the individual functioning of the child but this must be considered within the context of the family and others who form part of a child's daily life. In the same way, the mental health team itself must fit into the broader network of professionals working with the child and family. It is important to be clear what the specific work of the mental health team is, and how this will fit into the care plan which will be delivered and managed by a core group of professionals, often over-viewed by a case conference group.

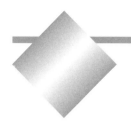

Postscript

A number of months went by without any news of Amber then, just before the Christmas of the year she left, there was a meeting with her social worker. The social worker chaired a meeting that the child psychiatrist attended and she said that Amber had settled in well with her grandparents. Amber had been able to see her brother and sister when their foster family took them on holiday in the south of England; a day out had been arranged at the local leisure complex. Amber was finding school a little difficult and she did not have any close friends, but her grandparents had encouraged her to join both the Brownies and the Red Cross group.

It was not until the following Christmas that we heard of her again. I was walking down the main corridor when I saw Amber's named nurse talking with a tall, graceful-looking girl whom I half recognized. She smiled at me and I recognized her as Amber. She was visiting her siblings and foster family and had asked if she could come to the unit. 'Everything is smaller than I remember,' she said, in a southern accent, her Geordie accent long gone. Her named nurse asked if there was anything Amber wanted to do while she was visiting. Amber smiled and asked after a few of the children she had known. She continued speaking, despite a number of interruptions from staff who were pleased to see her, and told the staff who were with her about her achievements in swimming. She had recently represented her county in the under-12s section. She was the proud owner of a large tabby cat called Spice and she had a lot of friends. She giggled as she lowered her voice to tell her named nurse the name of her boyfriend. Her speech and manner were that of a well-adjusted 11-year-old. She wanted to look at her old classroom, and her teacher had found a few drawings she had left.

I said my farewells and wished her a merry Christmas. A few minutes later, when I was in the office, I saw her going into the green group.

Amber's grandparents had called in to see the child psychiatrist and told her that all was well with Amber. They had not pursued the referral to the local child psychiatry unit because they felt that the move and getting settled in her new home was something they needed to do as a family. They had been supported by the adoption and fostering unit. They noted that Amber occasionally mentioned the unit in Newcastle and when she did it was in a happy way. She had formed a wide circle of friends although she did not have any particularly close friendships, and she had developed into an able artist as well as a swimmer. Amber had a sensitive nature, and could sometimes be very aloof, but she had not given them any cause for concern. They were not concerned about her development and felt that she was making a reasonable adjustment to their home and 'getting on' with life.

Amber had brought a Christmas card for members of the unit staff and when the time came for her to leave a number of staff gathered to wave good bye and to wish the family the compliments of the season.

In Amber, we saw a damaged child emerge from the chrysalis into the butterfly she had imagined in her play. Through therapeutic inter-vention she was able to transcend the difficulties that had previously marred her development as an individual. Not all cases are as clear cut as Amber's. Even though therapy helps the individual cope with the traumas or difficulties in their lives, not everyone emerges from the darkness as Amber did. Some children continue to have difficulties and may require therapeutic intervention into adolescent or adult life. In this case, the butterfly had time to dry her wings before she continued on to the next stage of her development.

After Amber had gone from the unit the therapeutic team also had to move on and provide new therapeutic space for other children referred to child psychiatry. The cycle of change continues.

REFERENCES

Ainscough K, Telford R 1995 Nondirective play therapy and psychotherapy theory: never the twain shall meet? British Journal of Occupational Therapy. 58: 201–203

Axline V M 1989 Play therapy. Churchill Livingstone, Edinburgh

Barker P 1971 Basic child psychiatry. Granada Publishing, London

Bion W 1962 A theory of thinking. International Journal of Psychoanalysis. Vol 43

The Children Act 1989 HMSO, London

Davenport G 1989 An introduction to child development. Unwin Hyman, London

Erikson E 1965 Childhood and society. Penguin, Harmondsworth

Freud S 1915 The unconscious. No. 14 standard edition. Hogarth Press, London pp. 161–216

Winnicott D 1986 Home is where we start from. Pelican, Harmondsworth

FURTHER READING

Bettleheim B, Rosenfeld A 1993 The Art of the obvious: developing insight for psychotherapy and everyday life. Thames and Hudson, London

Bowlby J 1953 Child care and the growth of love. Pelican, Harmondsworth

Copley B, Forryan B 1987 Therapeutic work with children. Robert Royce, London

Hagedorn R 1996 Foundatons for practice in occupational therapy, 2nd edn. Churchill Livingstone, Edinburgh

Kolvin I, Garside R, Nicol A, MacMillan A, Wolstenholme F, Leitch I 1981 Help starts here. Tavistock Publications, London

Laplanche J, Pontalis J 1988 The language of psychoanalysis. Karnac Books, London

Stern D 1985 The interpersonal world of the infant. Basic Books, New York

Winnicott D 1971 Playing and reality. Pelican, Harmondsworth

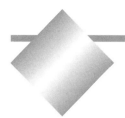

Index